LOVING LIFE
IN
RETIREMENT

LOVING LIFE
IN
RETIREMENT

Making Your New Freedom Work

Marvin H. Berenson M.D.

Cove Books
Palos Verdes Estates, California

Cove Books
Palos Verdes Estates,
California

For information:
Please contact Cove Books PVE@aol.com.

ISBN: 0-9700885-5-8

Library of Congress Control Number: 2009906081

Cover Design: Sam Wall

Printed in the United States of America

I dedicate this book to my loving partner,

Irene Cole Berenson

who has brought passion, excitement, romance and unending love into my life. Her positive feelings about life fill this book.

CONTENTS

PAGES FOR IMAGERY EXERCISES 1

ACKNOWLEDGEMENTS 5

A LETTER TO MY READERS 7

INTRODUCTION 13

Chapter 1:   OVERCOMING OBSTACLES 19

Chapter 2:   THE QUEST FOR LOVE 41

Chapter 3:   BARRIERS TO LOVE 61

Chapter 4:   FINDING ROMANCE 81

Chapter 5:   IGNITING YOUR SEX LIFE......................90

Chapter 6:   THE AGE FACTOR 126

Chapter 7:   THE PARENT-CHILD LINK.....................137

Chapter 8:   THE PATH TO SPIRITUALITY.................155

Chapter 9:   CREATIVITY FOR SENIORS 167

Chapter 10: EXPLORING YOUR INNER SELF 205

Chapter 11: DIET, EXERCISE AND HEALTH 231

Chapter 12: FILLING THE GAPS 261

Epilogue: FINAL AFFIRMATIONS 269

Addendum No. 1: PERSONAL GUIDE FOR

                CHANGING YOUR LIFE:

A TWELVE WEEK PROGRAM..................................... 271

Addendum No. 2: GUIDED IMAGERY EXERCISE 287

Addendum No. 3: INTRODUCTION TO
                 MENTAL IMAGERY...................... 292

ABOUT THE AUTHOR.. 307

PAGES FOR IMAGERY EXERCISES

1. Knowing your inner self....................................24

2. Symptom reduction 27

3. Understanding symptoms 28

4. Meditation 34

5. The Rag Doll Technique 66

6. Changing negative mindsets 67

7. Life as a loving person 68

8. Loving others...71

9. Loving 75

10. Enhancing your sex life

       Mutual pleasuring.......................................98
       Genital stimulation 101
       Intercourse...104
       The ways of romance...............................111
       Oral sex..114
       Tantric sex 117

11. The inner sanctuary......................................146

12. Saying good-bye to envy 159

13. Becoming spiritual.......................................160

14. Overcoming writer's block 181

15. Confronting your creative blocks 182

16. Writing from visual images 183

17. Imagery to stop wasting time 185

18. Overcoming procrastination 186

19. Inner growth—swallow a seed 186

20. Changing body parts 187

21. Changing your image 187

22. Changing your age 188

23. Breaking out of your mental prison 189

24. Freedom from paralysis 190

25. Encased in ice 191

26. Fighting the restrictive part of the self 191

27. Write a story 193

28. Draw a picture 194

29. Creating a drama 195

30. Overcoming creative blocks by role-playing ... 201

31. Assuming the identity of a master artist 201

32. Expanding your mind through fantasies 202

33. Image away your fears 215

34. Overcoming depression 217

35. Expressing anger 218

36. Overcoming a gambling obsession 221

37. Inferiority and gambling.............................. 222

38. Resolution of gambling compulsion............... 222

39. Tension headaches 224

40. Fighting migraine headaches 225

41. Headaches and anger................................... 226

42. Headaches and guilt 226

43. Overcoming insomnia: Falling asleep 228

44. Awakening in middle of night........................ 229

45. Maintaining a healthy heart.......................... 229

46. Overcoming fears of having a stroke 229

47. Compulsive eating: The refrigerator 250

48. Compulsive eating: The cupboard 250

49. Compulsive eating: The dining table 250

50. Blocking entrance to the food market............ 253

51. Blocking buying food in food markets 254

52. Compulsive eating at parties......................... 255

ACKNOWLEDGEMENTS

Many individuals contributed to bringing *Loving Life in Retirement* to fruition. First and foremost are the many patients, unable to make their retirement work, who entered therapy with me. I am grateful to them for providing me the background and understanding to write this book.

Without doubt *Loving Life in Retirement* would not exist in its present form, and possibly might not exist at all, but for the constant help from Irene, my wife. I owe her a deep debt of gratitude for her constancy in making me strive for excellence. With love and devotion she supported my desire to create this guide to enhanced living. She was my major editor, grammar expert and assistant and was pivotal in the direction and shape this book has taken.

Through his encouragement and inspiration Dr. Greg L. Finch, Associate for Collaborative Projects at Washington National Cathedral, became the spirit behind this book. His advice, which he freely gave throughout the writing, was always timely and helpful. I owe a deep sense of gratitude to him.

I am grateful to psychologist and friend, Dr. Helana Barry, who helped edit my book during the final phase of its development and was always available for advice. Her outrageous sense of humor embedded in her frequent emails certainly made writing this book easier and fun.

I'm also indebted to our own combined family for their constant support and readiness to help in whatever way needed. They include my three children: Renee, Doug and Alex and my three step-daughters: Vivian Cole, Yvonne Herron and Wendy Pratt. Our six children were all helpful but I especially want to acknowledge Wendy's readiness to edit, evaluate and critique parts of the manuscript and to offer unlimited support whenever needed. Doug, also constantly offered his unique insights adding new points of view during the writing of the book for which I'm grateful. I also owe many thanks to Wayne Herron and Steve Pratt, my two step sons-in-law for their wise input.

Four of our grandchildren, Kendra, Hayley, Jake and Justin offered valuable advice and evaluation of certain areas where their youthful insight proved useful. I learned that no one is too old to gain new insights from the very young.

I also want to deeply thank Don and Fran Shellgren, Maxine Kardell, Cindy Stokes, Susan O'Connor, BJ Golik, Mary Gene Slaven, Bob and Judy Geminder, Jean Tilem. Ruth Kisner , and Louise Wood who generously and unhesitatingly offered help when asked. I'm very grateful for their assistance.

I am very appreciative to Chuck Hurewitz for his clarity and suggestions in a wide variety of issues during the latter period of the book's development.

Finally, I've come to the last person who has played a pivotal part of this book, my book cover designer, Samantha (Sam) Wall. I owe her a deep sense of gratitude for creating a cover that truly speaks for me. Her creativity was only matched by her complete selflessness in time and effort as we collaborated on bringing the cover to life.

I also want to acknowledge my debt to many others who helped me directly or indirectly who, though nameless, are not forgotten.

A LETTER TO MY READERS

Preface

At breakfast, Irene, my wonderful wife and editor, looked at me squarely in the eyes holding up the copy of the latest version of my bio, with editing marks and suggestions to improve it. Quietly, but with a convincing smile, she said, "Marv, this just doesn't tell people who you are, the kind of person you are, how your sense of humanity has guided your life and led you into a field where you were completely dedicated to help people live better. People need to know that your book is you. It contains your lifelong efforts to maintain a healthy living style. You have never stopped exercising as long as I've known you. How many times have I heard you say that the true elixir of life is maintaining mental and physical fitness? Your youthfulness comes from the unending mental and physical activities that you do.

"I've watched as you so easily let your mind conjure up new images that feed your creativity. I've come to believe you when you say that anyone can do anything as long as they exclude comparisons with others. Anyone can paint or compose music at some meaningful level. Your constant striving to make your creative self more alive is a wonder to behold. I've never known anyone so imbued in the belief that anyone can be creative and always feel youthful and alive. You want to leave a legacy and you wrote a marvelous book. You need to let people know that you've lived everything in it. It all comes from your heart. Why don't you write them a letter?"

Dear Reader,

I'm sitting quietly and peacefully at my computer, reflecting on the words that I'm about to write you. They will be the first that you read of my new book. I wrote *Loving Life in*

Retirement to share with you the knowledge, insight and experience that I have accumulated in 83 years of living, teaching and practicing as a psychiatrist. I truly hope that what I have written will help guide you to a wonderful retirement. I know in my heart that all retirees can find new directions, increasing satisfaction and happiness. I filled my book with as much information as I could to provide the ways for you to create what you want in your life. Everyone should have dreams and do everything possible to fulfill them.

As a psychiatrist I have helped hundreds of older patients overcome barriers that stood in their way of a happy and meaningful life. Many felt lost and depressed after leaving their jobs. They lacked a sense of purpose. As they overcame their negative mindsets and changed how they thought, they grew and flourished. They saw the opportunity they had to create a new life. They came to understand the path to change that you too can take.

Anything is possible. Everyone can live a better life, a happier life, a more peaceful life.

I have always believed that we came into this world for a purpose. To accomplish whatever lies in our future we need to maintain our mental and physical health. I can't overemphasize the importance of keeping our bodies healthy and vital for they house our minds and souls; they are the repository of all our experiences, feelings, beliefs and hopes. Mental and physical health are paramount to all that we accomplish.

As I grew older and slowly overcame my own personal conflicts and continued to search for new ways for growth, I came to believe that "growing older never means becoming older." In a way as we grow older we are increasing our sense of youthfulness. We learn to simplify our lives and direct our energy to what matters. We learn how important it is to love and care for others but to not forsake ourselves in the process.

Self-love becomes necessary to create an inner sanctuary that nourishes our souls. We need to believe in our inner good and by so doing believe in our capacity to change. We see it about us. Everyone grows through change. Children do most of all, but older people are a close second. At our age we have shed the shackles of the past years and have a new freedom to explore entirely new lifestyles.

Writing this book at my age is not to be seen as unusual. I'm only 83 by the reckoning of a calendar. In real terms I'm ageless. The old adage that you are as old as you feel is true and attainable. Certainly I've slowed up a bit and my memory may not be as sharp as when I was 40 or 50 but I compensate with greater wisdom and understanding. Someday, when I pass away, I will still not be old. Dying only means that I've come to the end of my life cycle. It's the eternal sleep.

I know that we can all change and grow. I deeply believe that. I speak with the hope that all who read this book are motivated to change their lives. It wasn't by chance that the subtitle states. "Making Your New Freedom Work." In retirement we do have a new freedom but change doesn't come by chance. Many of you will have worked hard to become who you are, much as I did. You worked to constantly improve your life. Thus entering retirement was relatively easy and experienced as a continuance of your exciting and productive lifestyle. For those who haven't yet attained that level of satisfaction and want to become more creative, sexual, healthy and loving, this book will help you. I know it will. My heart is in it and I want it to become part of who you are. Always remember that retirement is just another name for a time period but in no way does it define you.

When I recently retired from private psychiatric practice and from my position as Clinical Professor of Psychiatry at the USC Keck School of Medicine, I never thought I was losing something. I loved teaching and watching the glowing faces of young psychiatrists grow into maturity knowing they would be giving back as they helped future patients. I gave of myself to them and added to the knowledge they accumulated from all their teachers. Now I want to give to you. Don't short change yourself. Believe fully in your ability to overcome all obstacles that impede your growth.

You can do it. My perpetual sense of youthfulness and aliveness that continue to permeate my exciting life can be yours.

It matters not what you decide to do. What matters is the attitude toward what you are doing and what you are feeling. Retirement becomes a time of transitions, one or many; each adds to your growing lifestyle. Sometimes new ideas pop into your head and become your current activity. Other ideas are in the planning stage for months and years. I thought about a book for retirees for several years before actually sitting down to write it. I saw the need for a book that would encompass the ideas, mental imagery techniques and exercises that I've so successfully used with myself and with countless others. Creativity would be the heart of the book. The subject is vast but for each individual it narrows down to the uniqueness of each of us. I borrowed heavily from a course in creativity that I gave for a number of years to small groups as well as from adapting the methods that induced my patients to become more creative. Other subjects so essential to our having a full life fell easily into the chapters that comprise this book. Everything I know to help people is here.

I don't want to end this letter without stating, actually pleading, that you avail yourself of every opportunity to change your life into what you most desire. My book is only one source of the wealth of information that waits for your discovery. The world is open. See the potential. See the vistas. Look beyond the horizon. Stretch your limbs and mind. A new world waits for you. Enter it.

Warmest wishes for your future,

Marvin Berenson

Twenty years from now, you will be more disappointed by the things you didn't do than by the ones you did do.
Explore. Dream. Discover.

—Mark Twain

*We must learn to reawaken and keep ourselves awake,
not by mechanical acts, but by an infinite expectation of the
dawn, which does not forsake us even in our soundest sleep.*

—Henry David Thoreau

*There is a vitality, a life force, an energy, a quickening that is
translated through you into action and because there is only
one of you in all of time, this expression is unique. And if you
block it, it will never exist through any other medium and be
lost.*

—Martha Graham

*Change and growth also start from within us. We can use
our mind's eye to imagine our lives as we would like them to
be. Our imagination can be a powerful motivating force to
enrich and transform our lives.*

—Eudora Welty

INTRODUCTION

For decades, as a psychiatrist, I treated many older adults as they faced the complex world of retirement. I watched them come to grips with obstacles that interfered with their desire to have a vital, happy life. Some were burdened by growing old, believing they would soon lose their physical and mental abilities. Others lacked passion about life and had opted out of most, if not all, activities. They often lost a sense of purpose and withdrew from society. Boredom and depression moved many to seek help. They looked into a dreary future and wondered what's so exciting about retirement.

Singly and as a group they asked, "What do I do now? Where do I turn for help? I don't want to live this way. I retired hoping to make a new life and I don't know how to do it."

Through our work they taught me what they needed and what direction I could take to help them. Slowly the ideas that fill this book took shape and developed into a clear and fundamentally new way to think about retirement. These individuals became the inspiration for this book.

Meanwhile, I was growing into that same age period and applied much of what I learned to myself. I decided that my retirement was not going to have anything to do with growing old. I was going to remain perpetually young. I was going to follow the dictates of my heart and live an exciting and fulfilled life. I would find the venues and activities to become truly alive.

What do those words mean? Becoming truly alive? As the old saying goes, 'When you feel it, you have it. And you know it.' Over many years I learned that what must be done, and I can only repeat, *must be done,* is to change your thinking and your mental attitude about growing old and about retirement. Everyone can do it. Many patients did it. I did it and you can do it.

And you can do it despite the present economic downturn that has affected our country. Many seniors now face economic hardships that may diminish their anticipated financial security. Instead of having the freedom to freely explore the world and live with minimal concern for their financial welfare, they believe their lives must be curtailed. Nothing can be further from the truth.

Certainly you may have to eat out less and take less expensive vacations and buy fewer things. But this in no way should interfere with finding the peace and happiness you desire. Whatever you have lost is gone. It is the past. You need to overcome any residual belief that your life is now impoverished. It isn't and won't be. You haven't lost your spirit and the inner belief in your personal integrity. You must not become a victim of conditions that are now mainly out of your control. You need to believe that you can and will rise above any temporary impoverishments through the power of your own thinking. This book will present you with many ideas and techniques to overcome any negative mental attitudes.

This change in our country and indeed the world's economic stability does not need to impinge upon your individual life. You can still utilize all the resources available to you to find that unique path you seek. Times like these can try men's souls but they also provide the impetus for you to make your senior years the best period of your life.

This is the time to learn new ways to expand your world. You will learn simple but very effective mental imagery techniques that will help you change. They are the same kind of mental imagery methods that famous athletes and actors use. I have simplified how to apply them. There are several ways to best use the exercises described in this book. You can practice any of the exercises and follow the ideas from any of the chapters that appeal to you or you can follow the twelve week program listed as Addendum No. 1. During a period of twelve weeks you will learn a realistic method that will lead to a revitalization of your life.

In Addendum No. 2 you will have an opportunity to take a guided imagery tour to enjoy the new power of your creative imagination.

By avoiding pitfalls, facing and overcoming barriers and never faltering in your search, you can create a new life. Your objective is to become a highly creative, vital, happy and self-directed person.

This book will help you make certain that such a scenario happens.

Love is an essential part of everyone's life, and especially for seniors. I discuss love in depth and suggest ways to help you seek out new sources of love and to maintain and enhance the love you already have.

The myth of sex for the young alone is put to rest. The enjoyment of sex is for everyone and older people can attain the many pleasures and the intimacy that accompanies it. Sex is fun and is certainly part of the pleasure that retired people should have. One chapter is a sex manual for finding heightened satisfaction and gratification in all your sexual desires. You will find all you need to know in enjoying sexuality as a senior. It's all here.

In the second half of life, people have entered a new area of consciousness and often seek spirituality and even a renewal of religion; I look at this delicate and essential subject with reverence. Although many people enter retirement already spiritual and sensitive to the elevation of the soul, many do not. The quest for spirituality concerns love, its connection to religion and believing in the goodness of self and the world around.

I don't lessen the importance of the many problems that all seniors face as they get older, such as sickness, injury and the aging of the body and mind. By developing a truly positive mindset about living well and happily you will better learn to handle the medical and psychological problems that confront all of us. And facing the end of your life cycle and the inevitability of death will be easier when you know that you are living as fully as possible.

You can actually become or even remain younger physically with proper diet and exercise programs. It's important to know that weight control is within your grasp no matter what difficulties you have faced in the past. It's less a matter of losing weight than how you feel about your body. Many times by changing your understanding of what dieting means you will discover that suddenly you can lose weight and keep it off. I include an uncomplicated but effective diet and weight control program that I've used successfully with hundreds of patients. It's based on several innovative ways to eat and diet and also on the use of imagery exercises.

Another area that many seniors avoid is exercise. Exercise should be like eating meals. A necessity. It's not whether you should exercise. You need to do it to maintain health and the feeling of youthfulness. It doesn't even have to take much time. But when you learn to like it you'll have another part of your life that gives you pleasure. And it's not as difficult or as time consuming as you might believe. You only have to change your thinking and it becomes feasible and an important and pleasant part of your life. When I take long walks or go to the gym I love the freedom of movement and the time for reflection.

Growing Younger: George, A case study

Simple things like changing your perspective about walking can make retirement more fun. One young man, George, 76, told me during his last therapy session what was the most important thing that he had learned from me. From emptiness and aloneness his life was now filled with so much that he smiled as he laughingly complained that he now needs to find a way to slow down. In the short time of two months he had become a published poet.

With a sly smile he asked if I recalled what I had told him about his attitude about hating to walk for exercise, much less for fun. He was a loner and walking seemed to add to his isolation. Although I did recall it, I asked him to remind me. "You told me," he said, "that no one is ever alone when he walks. You have your thoughts to accompany you, birds fly about and sing to you. Flowers are everywhere and the allure of roses beckons you to stop and smell the fragrance. Clouds present an ever-changing panorama. Saying 'good morning' to other walkers always elicits a smile."

Once George tried this new way of thinking about walking his life began to change. He now walks where the birds sing and where beautiful flowers peer from flower beds that surround every home he passes. Trees wave at him and the clouds hum briskly along making faces at him. He became so enamored by all he now saw that he decided to write poetry about his walks and everyday he does just that.

One day he shared some of his poems with a friend who showed them to an editor of the local newspaper. When one of his poems appeared in the newspaper George knew that he had truly grown younger. He was like a vibrant kid walking the streets looking for sources of material for his poems. Because of his personal inclinations he preferred to walk alone, surrounded by the ever changing panorama of the neighborhood and excited by all the new places he found to walk. He walked everywhere and wrote what he felt, saw and had become.

Reaching 65 is a promise made by your body that you may well have another twenty or thirty years of life ahead. Imagine twenty to thirty years of retirement. My objective is to help you take advantage of that time and to make your later years highly productive and gratifying.

Can we change our minds?

Can you change your mind to accomplish what you want? The simple answer is YES. To help you reach that goal I included in this book every kind of mental exercise that I believed would benefit seniors.   There are fifty-two exercises. You may not have time to use all of them but you will have many to select from. Best of all, I encourage and show how you can develop your own imagery exercises in any areas that you want. Do you want to write, be an artist, a gardener, make films, take pictures, write screen plays, sculpt, make pots, cook, go back to school, learn a new profession, improve your relationships with family and friends, overcome inner fears and doubts, learn tricks for dieting or improve yourself? The answers are here and the exercises are clear; they offer examples of ones that you can use or they show you how to create your own.

During this time creativity stands high. Creativity is inherent in everyone and as seniors you can rediscover your own. It comes from stirring up your inner curiosity and taking advantage of your new sense of freedom. Think back upon your childhood. Remember your laughter and glee when you discovered the wiggling nose of a rabbit or the purring of a contented kitten. Or having an open field to run and explore. Think back on your earliest discoveries of science in the guise of games—blowing bubbles, watching a balloon rise swiftly into the sky or the magic of pictures on a television screen.

Changing your mindsets, removing all negative thoughts, anything that interferes with moving into your senior years with hope and the knowledge that you can make it a wonderful time of your life is what this book is about. Better still, you can make this the best time of your life. Is this possible? You bet it is. I've seen it with hundreds of patients and friends. No one needs to be left in the doldrums or left out. You can be one who flies and sings and dances as you grow younger.

It is now time to reawaken your inner zest for newness and exploration. It has not been lost but is merely lying dormant waiting to be animated by a new sense of vitality. You want to enjoy these years through new and ever inquisitive eyes. There is no limit to what you can do or experience.

Growing old is really a version of growing young. Aging is a gift, an opportunity to fly high, walk in the clouds, soar in your imagination and accomplish unheard of dreams. It's all up to you.

So come along with me. The journey will be worth your time and I'll certainly hold a candle to help light your way. The world awaits you.

Chapter One

OVERCOMING OBSTACLES

We do not quit playing because we grow old; we grow old because we quit playing.

—Oliver Wendell Holmes

It is always in season for the old to learn.

—Aeschylus

"I did it. I finished my first 10K," Jim shouted, as he rushed into his wife's waiting arms. Jim was 74 on that special day.

"That's quite beautiful," the young teacher said, as she looked at Anne's new painting. "I remember when you started this class six weeks ago you told me that you had never painted in your life. It's wonderful what you have accomplished." Anne was 67 as she beamed at her still life painting of glistening apples and lemons bursting forth from a colorful bowl placed on a table.

"I'm so glad I decided to come over and say hello. I was so nervous," Ralph murmured to Gloria, a young woman of 81 who had just put her arm in his as they walked out of the restaurant. Ralph was 86. He smiled as he thought back to three hours ago when he had approached Gloria.

"What a great meal. Is this really the very first meal that you cooked?" Cindy asked, giving Robert a hug. "Never knew you had it in you." Robert was 77.

"I've always wanted to play the piano," Carol said quietly to the young piano teacher who smiled warmly as he watched his new pupil sit down before her piano. Carol was 89.

What do these voices have in common? All are from seniors who had previously felt alone, unfulfilled and dreading their continued existence as they moved into their older years. They are the voices that will guide this book: people who found new ways to make life vital and meaningful, more productive and creative. They went from friendlessness to sharing their lives with others. These people found new love, activities that gave them satisfaction, and better communication with their children and grandchildren. They felt joy and clapped their hands in glee as they explored a new and wonderful world. The senior world had finally opened its arms and welcomed them into its grasp.

A COMMON THEME

Jim, Anne, Ralph, Robert and Carol had not always faced the daunting years of retirement with such ease and evident happiness. Instead they had faced obstacles that seemed insurmountable and finally in quiet desperation had sought counseling and therapy. They and many other seniors, unable to find solutions to overcome the barriers that prevented them from leading a fruitful and satisfying life, came to see me for guidance. This book is the result of what I have learned from them and the ways that I helped them find the new life they sought. It is a compilation of what I believe it takes to lead seniors to a more satisfying and creative life as older people than what most had experienced previously, even when younger.

People confront their senior years with varying degrees of confidence and hope. Some make the transition from work to retirement easily, having prepared for this new period of life. For them retirement is actually a temporary period when they transition from one type of work or activity to another already planned. Whether they call the new activity a hobby, avocation, another vocation or work makes no difference. It's a matter of having something pleasurable and satisfying to do after retiring.

A lack of planning, financial difficulties, health problems, emotional conflicts about aging, as well as unresolved mental conflicts, can be impediments to finding fulfillment and contentment in retirement. Boredom, unhappiness and even despair can result.

Whether a person retires because of company policy, illness or by self-determination, many of the same challenges exist. They include maintaining good health, finding satisfying activities, improving relationships with family and friends, discovering spiritual meaning in their final years and dealing with the prospect of death.

For those without a plan for occupying their newfound time there is a need to explore various activities and arrive at one or more that will suit their needs and personality. I call this group the **explorers.**

Entering the retirement period as an explorer can be exciting and rewarding. There is freedom to evaluate unlimited new areas that have the potential to markedly expand your life. To take full advantage of this exploratory period you need to assess your mental and physical abilities to best direct your path. It is important to be able to develop the resources to pursue your dreams.

Becoming a successful retiree depends on developing and maintaining a positive attitude about life and yourself and doing all you can to improve your mental and physical health.

WHAT ARE OUR OBSTACLES?
(Brandon's Story)

What are the specific obstacles that many retirees face that need to be carefully assessed and then changed? A rather typical patient, let's call him **Brandon**, was a 67 year-old, tall, ruggedly good-looking man who entered therapy with a litany of complaints. Life, after two years of retirement, did not prove to be fun at all.

As an executive VP of a large corporation, his previous life had been planned and satisfying. All that had changed. Without the exciting repartee with business associates and planned business travel or interesting lunch dates with attractive women and inspiring colleagues, he floundered in boredom and inactivity. Initially he had tried everything that could conceivably stimulate him. Golf, tennis, bridge, education classes, painting, charitable work, joining a gym, Internet dating, hiking with the Sierra Club and senior citizen clubs. Nothing worked. He became depressed, gained weight and withdrew.

Does this sound familiar? Many seniors who try to adapt to retirement face similar issues with comparable results. Retirement has become a battleground of one obstacle after another. Instead of finding the hoped for satisfaction there is usually a gradual decay of interests, enthusiasm and zeal. Initial attempts to find activities for the hoped for gratification fail and a growing and persistent negativism and pessimism ensue. Retirement has become a one-way street to emptiness and depression.

Seniors succumb to preoccupation with illnesses, the inevitable loss of friends and family, and a belief that they are declining physically and mentally. In other words, the prospect of a wonderful and exciting world to spend one's final years has evolved into its opposite. My efforts will be directed to giving you the tools and knowledge to not only make certain such a scenario does not develop for you, but to give you the methods to climb new mountains of successful living during your retirement period.

Negative Mindsets

Brandon believed he had tried everything, even meditation and yoga, and felt there was something wrong with him. In a sense he was right, as he soon discovered. Through no fault of his own he had developed negative mindsets and beliefs that interfered with his being able to take advantage of activities that would normally be satisfying. What he learned and used to transform his life can be easily grasped and used by anyone who needs new insights and directions as they enter this new phase of life.

Boredom

Boredom is frequently one of the first clues retirees get that retirement is not working. For people who rarely felt bored before retiring the symptom is more telling and should be viewed as a possible important indicator of early withdrawal and negativism. When attempts to find that wonderful path leading to an active and fulfilling life fail, the retiree becomes frustrated and eventually defeated. Boredom results. Frequently a precursor and often an adjunct to depression, boredom may have become a major impediment that prevents people from finding new interests and resuming old ones.

Resuming old interests, actively pursuing a new activity, getting involved in sports, reading, anything to overcome boredom are the antidotes. Don't wait until boredom has developed into depression before striving to change your lifestyle. Don't let negative habit patterns, fears, lack of direction or inadequate understanding of the process of retiring interfere with your making retirement into a truly special time of your life.

When you're feeling stymied or depressed and becoming increasingly negative, the first step to changing will be to ask yourself why you're in that particular state of mind. Directing attention to our mental states and attempting to overcome any negative mindset frequently sets us on the path to recovery. For most people there is no need to consult a therapist for guidance. Instead, learning methods to reduce symptoms and becoming more self-directed can lead to self-improvement.

During the course of reading this book you will learn various techniques that will facilitate your search for self-improvement and overcoming negative mindsets. Like climbing a mountain you first must remove all obstacles that prevent you from gaining access to the paths leading to its summit. We begin with the strong emphasis on getting rid of all negativity and adopting a very positive attitude about your future. With that in mind here are three exercises that will foster this intent.

EXERCISE NO. 1: KNOWING YOUR INNER SELF

Sit in a comfortable chair. Close your eyes. Take several deep breaths and feel your body relax. Now breathe normally. Visualize your entire body relaxing and feel tension draining from your mind, as well as your body.

Turn your attention inwardly, into your inner self. To enter this part of yourself imagine seeing yourself walking along a mountain path. You look out on a beautiful canyon. Birds are flying everywhere. You come to a plateau and see a cave, a symbol of your inner self. Enter the cave. It is permeated by a soft light. You know that you are entering some deeper, hidden part of yourself and have an opportunity to discover many things. Let your imagination soar; feel free, don't hesitate and don't hide.

Be attentive to whatever your mind is revealing. Just let it happen. Look at the walls of the cave. Notice whatever is on them. Proceed further into the cave following a narrow tunnel. You will come to a large cavern. In the middle is a massive stone. Seated on it is an old man who you soon learn is very wise. Introduce yourself to him and ask him any questions that appear in your mind. His answers may astonish you. When you are finally ready to leave, thank him for being there for you and ask him if you can return in the future. Then leave the cavern, return to the plateau and go back down the path. Feel contented and know that you have taken the first step in your journey into a new future.

For now there is no need to try to analyze what you're experiencing. Just enjoy it. After five to ten minutes open your eyes and acknowledge the satisfaction of having made

contact with a part of yourself that you want
to know better.

This exercise introduces you to becoming more introspective. Practice as frequently as you want. Becoming tuned into yourself will facilitate your benefiting from other exercises that are gradually introduced. Enjoy this brief period of relaxation and your evolving self-intimacy.

There are many ways to reach the inner you. Some people prefer to open a door to an unknown world or go underwater or into a dense forest to reach their inner self. They face whatever they discover. Your imagination will guide you.

THE TIME TO RETIRE

If you are able to retire whenever you desire always carefully question why you selected a particular time. Early or very late retirement has meaning. Are you running away from work that has become boring, dissatisfying or too difficult? Some people feel they are failing in their work and leave before it's noticed or sometimes they are on the verge of being fired and take an easier way out. Such feelings need to be carefully evaluated before these individuals give up work that otherwise might be rewarding and even creative.

If you delay retirement, are you doing it because of love for your job, or do you believe you're unable to retire because of financial needs or fear of the unknown? Or do you fear depression or loneliness?

Frequently you make the right choice but at other times the choice may backfire, especially when you choose early retirement. Today when seniors live into their eighties and nineties they need to find meaningful activities that will fill these many years. At times your work is the most desirable occupation or, at least, it's a known method for maintaining pleasure and satisfaction as you age. At other times, early retirement truly opens the door to new and more exciting vocations. Time opens up and you can walk into a new world.

FEARS OF AGING

Fear of dying frequently plays a pivotal part in a person's inability to enjoy retirement. None of us knows when our time is up, but allowing fears of dying to dominate our thinking is tantamount to giving up on life. To remain healthy careful medical evaluation of all symptoms, treating potential illnesses that may shorten life and the use of preventative medical programs are essential.

As we get older, friends and relatives will be dying, which tends to intensify one's fears of death. It's much better to accept the inevitability of death as the final stage in our grand life cycle. Fears do not need to be part of our natural life cycle. Instead put your resources to work to make your life fulfilling and highly satisfying. To enjoy retirement we need to minimize and hopefully eliminate these fears. No older person should live with such concerns. The need to accept the inevitability of death is necessary to reduce anxiety; however, most important is living as healthfully as possible.

New symptoms of illness can be a cause of some concern. Our slowly ebbing resistance to illness and the breakdown of our immune defenses, all part of growing older, can lead to new medical problems. You should consider the possibility of emotional difficulties as the cause when you have eliminated organic/medical disorders. Unless symptoms are clearly due to an acute or chronic medical problem, you should consider other reasons, such as, changes in your environment, with your family or friends or new worries about growing older may now be producing symptoms. Worry, anxiety, reactions to personal or world conditions can now be taking their toll. Symptoms are the result.

Believing that you're a healthy, vital person who has temporarily succumbed to some hidden emotional problem can quickly relieve you of the symptoms and also direct your attention and energy to the underlying causes of the emotional symptoms. Courage and believing in yourself are the ingredients that will guide you to overcome such conflicts. Medical needs and emotional conflicts need quick resolution to prevent them from becoming major obstacles to the enjoyment of your retirement.

If you are in any doubt about your ability to change your thinking and behavior patterns and eradicate your emotional symptoms you may benefit by experimenting with the following exercise. This exercise will help you overcome anxiety and apprehension about your future. Whatever is causing this anxiety you must face objectively and logically. Always keep in mind that imagery exercises are not a substitute for medical treatment or evaluation. All medical symptoms need medical clearance.

EXERCISE NO. 2: SYMPTOM REDUCTION

> Sit in a comfortable chair. Close your eyes. Take several deep breaths and feel your body relax. Now breathe normally. Visualize your entire body relaxing. Feel the tension draining from your mind, as well as your body. Focus on any symptoms that you feel are making you uncomfortable, less efficient, negative or disturbed in any way. If your symptom is anxiety or depression, try to connect these symptoms to underlying causes. Anxiety can appear as indigestion. Headaches can accompany depression. Stress in a relationship may be a factor in your symptoms. Face your symptoms while in a relaxed state.
>
> Convincingly repeat, "My symptoms will diminish as I go into a deeper state of relaxation. I will feel better. My pain will disappear. I am more relaxed. I am feeling better." Feel the quieting of your mind and body and the reduction of your symptoms. You must believe that your mind has the power to change your body and your thinking.

Later on I'll discuss more fully how to use special mental techniques to create imagery to help overcome your symptoms. For now these exercises are introductions to the use of your mind to change your thinking and behavior. Do them whenever you desire.

Facing an unknown world is always a bit scary. Everyone who goes through retirement encounters some anxiety, which makes facing retirement more difficult. Your objective is to find ways to change your fears, no matter how slight or how intense. Reducing and eventually conquering fears will enhance the process of change.

Becoming the vital and highly functioning person you want to be gets easier as your anxiety level decreases. Having a free, open minded and upbeat frame of mind will make everything you do more satisfying.

Retirement is a special time period when these inner changes can occur. It will change your life. The more you know yourself the greater the impetus to change. Self-knowledge is a wonderful tool that has many uses. Reflecting on your inner fears even as you come to know yourself better is a major step toward self-knowledge that ultimately will lead to overcome them.

The following exercise can augment the development of greater introspection. This time you'll try to discover the meaning behind feelings or symptoms that you have. This exercise will show you a new way to look at yourself that can lead to new insights. Doing these exercises can lead to changes in thinking that will, in turn, become a fundamental part of your transformation.

EXERCISE NO. 3: UNDERSTANDING SYMPTOMS

> Sit in a comfortable chair. Close your eyes. Take several deep breaths and feel your body relax. Now breathe normally. Visualize your entire body relaxing and feel tension draining from your mind, as well as your body. Focus on any symptoms that you currently have. Tell yourself that you want to better understand what the symptoms mean. Ask it to tell you the cause or meaning behind your symptoms. Listen closely to what you sense and "hear."

Trust yourself. Developing this kind of intimacy is highly rewarding.

Here is how one of my patients addressed this exercise. "I have a terrible headache. My head is on fire. I asked the fire why it's hurting me. The fire immediately turns into a fiery head and speaks to me. 'Because you were bad.' I'm baffled and ask it, 'How am I bad?' 'You scolded your daughter for something that she didn't do. You were angry at yourself and took it out on her.' 'I didn't mean to do it,' I cried out. 'But you did and you hurt her. You need to suffer.' 'What can I do?' 'Go to her and apologize.' 'I can't do that. It happened yesterday.' 'Yes you can. Do it now and tell her you were wrong. Apologize and tell her you love her.'"

Is this a typical example? Yes. This patient had ignored the need to apologize to his six year-old daughter until he did the exercise. Just be free with your imagination and it will guide you. Trust yourself.

If working with your mind is new to you take note that such exercises are useful and, if practiced over a period of time, can lead to insight, as well as mental and physical changes. We shall use similar techniques for different purposes during the course of this book. My purpose is to give you real tools that you can use for the rest of your life in a variety of ways that will facilitate the changes you seek.

These three related exercises can be used to just relax but if you desire to enhance your knowledge you must follow the exercises as described. It is important that you avoid expecting revelations, although some may come. By turning inward you are stimulating a type of self-growth that will definitely give you many dividends.

Never Give Up

As many retirees begin to seek new interests and activities they tend to approach them with enthusiasm, hope and often as an adventure. However, if obstacles appear or they begin to doubt their ability to achieve their dreams, fears and doubts can arise and their adventure may grind to a halt. In a sense their ongoing search may lead to periods of disruption as they try to deal with doubts and negative feelings. Instead of becoming an open minded and happy explorer they succumb to uncertainties and qualms. Some people tend to withdraw and give up the search for a new life. It is worth repeating that **your objective is to never give up the search** and to work to overcome all obstacles as you try out new interests. Only in this way can you truly arrive at that longed for life that offers so much potential satisfaction for your future.

RETIREMENT: A WORLD OF OPPORTUNITY

Retirement— I can't emphasize this enough—can be a time of great creativity, productiveness and newfound pleasures as you discover new activities and interests. With an almost unlimited number of appealing activities (to be discussed in a later chapter) part of your fun will be deciding what to pursue knowing that you are under no contract or obligation to continue anything. This is a time of freedom and exploration. And if you decide to take a period to rest or do essentially nothing no one but yourself, can interfere with your decision. Hopefully, the idea of finding new sources of pleasure will become too appealing to ignore.

Initially, many retirees narrow the list of interesting projects down to those that are most tempting and tackle them first. A surprising large number of retirees initially try playing sports. Physical activity of any sort is the primary way to keep your body and mind healthy and youthful. And it can be much fun and a potential vehicle for social interaction.

Three favorites are walking, golf and tennis. Many retirees intensify their interest in sports they had enjoyed playing as younger adults. Others pick up sports that they had loved as children and adolescents but had not been able to include in their life once they joined the work force and became parents. But as a retiree time is no longer restrictive. You are now free to pick and choose the activities that fill this period of your life.

As a senior, exercising will be like nourishment for the body and the mind. The easiest, and perhaps the most satisfying, is walking. Finding new areas to walk, either alone or with a friend or spouse, is especially satisfying. Daily walks alone can immeasurably improve your health.

Another physical activity that appeals to many seniors is joining a **gym**. Most fitness centers cater to all ages and welcome seniors to participate in all their exercise programs. For many seniors physical fitness becomes the center of their activities as they realize the positive effect it has on their mental and physical well-being.

Consider exercise as one of your continuing senior activities and keep in mind that you're not in a race to prove yourself to anyone.

SPORTS AND EXERCISE PROGRAMS

Sports and exercise programs can be among the most enjoyable and beneficial of the experiences available to seniors and as a bonus will generally create opportunities to meet new friends. They include:

- Tennis, doubles are especially beneficial and less stressful.
- Golf, definitely a worthy pursuit.
- Hiking which can open new terrains for exploration.
- Racquet ball can be vigorous. Need to pick your partner carefully.
- Bicycling offers a wide range of roads, parks and terrain.
- Yoga, with an instructor who encourages the students to go at their own pace.
- Sailing, very relaxing, especially on calm and balmy days.
- Tai Chi, good for balance and quieting the body and mind.
- Swimming for all around conditioning.
- Resistance exercises for strength building.
- Endurance exercise for cardiac fitness. Includes exercise bikes, treadmills, elliptical gliders, jogging and even stair masters.

- Softball. Senior leagues are available for playing this all-time favorite.
- Gardening. Has a wide range of ways to participate, but can be very satisfying.
- Setting up a home exercise program, including stretching and resistance training, can be highly rewarding.
- Aerobic classes in various fitness centers. Many are handled by instructors who advise participants to go at their own pace.

Many other activities are appealing to seniors and very satisfying. You know most of them but it may be worth my listing some of the more prominent as a reminder that much lies ahead of you. You only have to open the gates.

Writing can be extremely meaningful to seniors. Whether you prefer prose, poetry, essays, short articles, drama, plays, scripts, biography or humor, writing down your ideas can be illuminating, creative and fulfilling. Many seniors write autobiographical books to leave for their children and grandchildren. Others develop a great interest in writing and seek to publish their books. With the advent of Print on Demand methods it is extremely easy to publish a book.

Acting. Many acting classes, groups and theater venues exist for seniors. Did you ever want to act? Try it. Nothing to lose. At the least it will sharpen your awareness of how various actors perform. Look into the development of theater and movies. Much as writing sharpens your skills and helps you develop facility in evaluating books, acting enlivens your mind to the intricacies of acting and scripts.

Mental activities, in general, sharpen the mind and help you maintain your mental alertness and acuity. Card games, crossword puzzles, chess, bridge, various games, especially those you can play with your grandchildren are fun and brain exercisers..

Taking an active interest in environmental issues, politics, civic programs, teaching and participating in charities all help in filling this special time in your life.

In subsequent chapters we'll focus on these and other activities to clear your path of barriers that might interfere with developing your interests.

Remember Brandon? After trying unsuccessfully to make his retirement fun and meaningful, he gave up, fell into depression, gained weight and withdrew. How did Brandon find the solutions that would eventually transform his life? Although he had initially tried many activities before starting therapy he had quickly succumbed to his doubts and beliefs that nothing would really make a difference in his life. Overcoming this negative attitude was crucial for him to succeed in changing his life. So the pursuit of new interests now meant increasing his ability to explore his future with excitement and the belief he would be able to find what he sought. As he changed his negative attitudes Brandon became excited by the prospect of uncovering something new and stimulating. He began to view his future as one of new opportunities and saw retirement as an unparalleled period for discovery and growth.

Certainly, he was surprised to learn that as he grew older he could aspire to a higher level of awareness and productivity. He did not dismiss any activity, course or project as a possibility. Perhaps his ideas will offer you a new perspective. Trying activities that once seemed foreign or even esoteric can lead to an entirely new understanding of yourself and bring you new challenges and stimulation.

Brandon's desire to become more introspective led to a study of Eastern religions and meditation. After attending classes he focused on Buddhism and Zen. To his surprise he learned that there are many ways to meditate. He began his study of meditation by going to several retreats and to the Self-Realization Center in Los Angeles. Since I believe that practicing a form of meditation is beneficial for body and mind, I'll describe a simple, but highly effective form that you can practice now. To enter a deep state of relaxation you focus on a sound or mantra to focus or concentrate your mind.

For many it may become a devoted form of relaxation and a way to find inner peace when practiced daily over a period of time.

EXERCISE NO. 4: MEDITATION

> Sit in a comfortable chair. Close your eyes.
> Breathe normally. With each inhalation say to
> yourself the sound O while breathing through
> your nose. With each exhalation say to
> yourself the sound NA (pronounced nah) while
> breathing through your mouth (the nose can
> be used, if more comfortable). You will soon
> feel your entire body relax and the tension
> draining from your mind, as well as your
> body. Continue meditating for 15 to 20
> minutes while repeating the mantra O NA.

While experiencing meditation you must try to maintain a
passive state of mind. Try to control any tendency to think,
imagine, fantasize, question or other active thinking.
Whenever any other thought or distraction comes into your
mind merely return to the mantra- O NA. Don't question
what the distraction is –just return to the mantra. By this
passive approach you will enter and maintain an alpha
state of mind meaning that your brain waves are between 8
and 14 cycles per second, a state of high suggestibility and
mental quietness.

When your desired time period is up you merely open
your eyes. Although your time doesn't have to be exact you
can open your eyes while meditating and look at a clock
that you have placed in front of you without exiting the
alpha state, if you do not actively react to the time. Your
mind is familiar with time and thus merely opening your
eyes and looking at the clock remains a passive action.

During the first few weeks or longer, if desired, as part
of your meditation, I find it useful to silently express some
affirmation just before you open your eyes. Such words as,
"I will be wide awake and feel wonderful, fully alive and
joyful when I open my eyes." Or you may repeat an
affirmation to stimulate a positive mindset. For example,
you might repeat, "I am becoming more and more creative
or loving or adventurous." Or "I am no longer afraid of the

dark or driving at night." Affirmations can be changed at will to fit what you desire to accomplish.

THE PROCESS OF EXPANDING LIFE

From the desire to relax his mind and body, a major benefit from meditation, Brandon began to seek spiritual meaning and guidance. He met several new friends who were devoted to the pursuit of spiritual enlightenment and encouraged him to follow a similar path. Following this interest he tried several different types of Yoga and discovered that they improved his spiritual search. He finally settled on a Yoga class where the teacher quickly recognized each participant as separate and emphasized that each person progress according to individual needs and ability. Brandon was beginning to enjoy his own bodily and mental development and no longer measured his success by comparison to others. He was truly enjoying his individuality.

Wanting to give more to the natural world brought Brandon into the world of environmentalists. His zeal to protect the earth and the need to overcome the obstacles of both the government and business who, in his opinion, were dragging their feet in providing the kinds of protection the world needed, led him to assume a leadership role in several environmental organizations.

Although retired he decided to reenter the working world by becoming a consultant to various corporations that could benefit from the knowledge gained from his previous professional life. He learned that his age was not an impediment in seeking employment, but, rather in his case, a benefit. He could rely upon vast experience and wide knowledge of the corporate world to contribute to his value as a consultant and eventually connect to many people he had once known. His knowledge and experience were desired and sought.

He attended a course at the extension division of Santa Monica City College to study music and literature. He offered to teach a course in a local high school extension division on how to develop personal business plans for retirees who were concerned for their future financial security. His course quickly became popular and it was there that he met the woman who would eventually become his second wife. New friends came into his life with whom he felt intimate and close. His life had become full. He had become a vital and active older person.

When he ended therapy, he was looking forward to a vigorous and highly satisfying life. He no longer had doubts that his future would be the most gratifying period of his life. Brandon's journey is not unique. His is the story of many retirees and it can be yours.

REFLECTIONS

Brandon's improvement and future depended upon the same resilience and inner power that each of us has to overcome personal deficiencies. Our tools of self-awareness and self-exploration can open our minds to change. Brandon gave credibility to the underlying capacity we have to rise above most personal handicaps.

No matter what obstacles stand in the way, the time comes when we face the daunting, but exciting, time of seeking and selecting activities to fill our coming retirement. Emulating Brandon's decision to evaluate many interests before making his final selections will help lead retirees to fruitful and satisfying results. I suggest that all retirees follow a similar path. During the search you will broaden your views of your future and find new activities that will surprise and delight you and lead to a more fulfilling life.

It is less the type of activity you engage than the pursuit of pleasure in whatever you do. If sports greatly interest you, many venues exist to help fill that interest. You can become an active member of a team of seniors or join a club of like-minded enthusiasts. You can join other seniors who devote their time helping youngsters develop their skills in various sports. The same approach works for any interest, such as, academic pursuits, political agendas, travel, nature and environmental activities, creativity, writing, art and many others.

Fulfilling Dreams

> *Retirement is almost unlimited in its potential to fulfill long postponed dreams and gives us time to discover new dreams. As we get older, we reap the benefit of experience and knowledge, and can avoid many of our past mistakes. We are ready to take advantage of the opportunities ahead.*

What can interfere with your pursuing such dreams? Some retirees may be thwarted by deeper emotional problems, which might require therapy or counseling. At times, poor or inappropriate relationships may interfere with the pleasures and peace that can come with retirement. Holding on to grievances that diminish one's sense of self may become an obstacle. Most people, however, can overcome many of these psychological difficulties through self-understanding and a strong desire to change.

Symptoms, such as boredom, depression, loneliness, emptiness and obsessive doubts that relate to retirement, can usually be overcome as the efforts to enrich your retirement period begin and continue. Ways of overcoming such symptoms and barriers will be discussed more fully later.

Many prefer to seek new activities that suit their social needs, such as charities, book clubs and group dancing. Some prefer to explore their lives over a number of years, kind of like spreading the passage into retirement over a longer time span. Some believe retirement is a time for relaxation and prefer not to engage in new activities. Many retirees find such an existence fulfilling. However, even that group can find new ways to achieve a new sense of meaning in their lives.

There is no absolute formula that will satisfy all of us, but there are many preferred methods that can lead to fulfilling your dreams. We will examine many of them in future chapters. To facilitate your search and the exploration of this exciting period that lies ahead I would like to suggest that you **create a journal** that can act as a repository for experiences, activities and changes in your life.

In general, we have many years ahead that need to be filled with satisfaction. We are given an opportunity to make choices and are free to change, switch back and forth into several areas of work, not work at all, or find other ways to gain satisfaction. As older people have gained more political power the previous tendency to relegate seniors to a lesser social status has diminished. Age discrimination is disappearing. People can and do work into their late sixties, seventies and eighties. Even people living into their nineties can have productive and meaningful lives. It is our duty to remove any obstacles that interfere with this picture.

Relationship with Adult Children

One area that must be carefully assessed is your relationship with your adult children. The importance of improving relationships with your children, if needed, can't be overemphasized. The pleasures of having a warm and loving adult relationship with older children are without parallel. There is no other relationship that duplicates it and it should be sought by all parents. Without it many older people feel dissatisfied and unhappy and struggle to find real fulfillment in their later years.

Such relationships evolve out of the understanding and closeness initiated in childhood that continue throughout life. It is not something that you have to specifically target. It's a natural occurrence when parents and children love and respect each other. When it did not develop as desired then it behooves both parents and children to do whatever is necessary to establish such a connection. Having a full, open, honest and mutually satisfying relationship with adult children is attainable by most couples.   For   those who elected not to have children of their own, developing and maintaining a close connection to nieces, nephews and the children of older friends may also enhance life.

As we grow older we often resort to reminiscence to add spice and pleasure to our lives. Inherent in such recollection are the feelings of love and closeness to others.

Eliminate negativism, if possible, to help foster the intimacy that can become so important to the serenity and richness of our retirement years.

Resuming old Relationships

The period of retirement becomes an opportunity to make peace with significant persons from the past. This usually includes more than just parents. Think back to the relationships with grandparents, other close relatives and friends who have long disappeared. Consider those relationships that were ended or that have become distant and determine which bear reevaluation. Many times the reasons for the ending of former relationships are forgotten and only a vague negative feeling remains.

Would you benefit by attempting to reestablish these relationships? You are now embarking on a voyage of change and carrying the dark clouds of the past with you may impede your progress. There is value in cleaning out your mental cupboards. Whether you decide to resume the relationship or not is less important than ridding yourself of negative feelings and beliefs.

Some lifelong friendships provide a cushion of support not afforded by later friends and are an integral part of a full life. Unlike the benefits of maintaining a close and loving relationship with parents, friends often provide intimacy unavailable from family members. Good and intimate friends are among the treasures in life and old friends among the most rewarding of those treasures.

We enter our senior years hoping for new pleasures and satisfaction. We know that many years lie ahead for us, at least twenty on average when we reach 65. Time looms ahead as a beacon to draw us into a new era.

Can this become your most creative and vital period? I hope that, as you read on, you will find many ideas that help guide you to new adventures and discoveries.

> *Perhaps you will agree with me that*
> *the word retirement should be retired*
> *from our vocabulary, or, at the very*

least, we should change its meaning. Instead, think of revitalized and creative living, a time of opening your horizons, not closing them. It's a time of expanding your life knowing that in this final episode you will find the fulfillment you seek.

CONCLUSIONS

Retirement presents an opportunity to establish a vital, creative and fun-loving life. Instead of assuming that this period is fraught with obstacles and that you are in a declining period of life, see it as exciting, alive, and the time to forge new paths, discover new interests and make new friends. There are many steps you can take to prepare for retirement to help avoid some of the pitfalls that can trap retirees. Developing interests, accepting retirement as a new, exciting and welcomed stage of life sets your future in a positive framework. If you are entering this period of life and are uncertain what to expect or what to do, become an explorer and discover a new life. Instead of obstacles you will see your future filled with the lightness of life, the beauty of nature and the aliveness of your own mind.

Chapter Two

THE QUEST FOR LOVE

Let us cherish and love old age, for it is full of pleasure. The best morsel is reserved to the last.

—Seneca

There is more hunger for love and appreciation in this world than for bread.

— Mother Theresa

I did not know I loved you until I heard myself telling so, for one instance I thought, "Good God, what have I said?" and then I knew it was true.

— Bertrand Russell

Love—that word of wonder and magic. When it's in our life, we fly. When it eludes us we sink. When it is neither here nor there, merely elusive and often scurrying just out of reach, we are tantalized and frustrated.

Love can be part of everyone's life, no matter what age. It fills and nourishes

> *us. It helps make us bountiful and giving. It puts a glow on our face and a fire in our hearts. Our life and world become more vital. Above all else, we want to have love in our retirement years. Yet, many face retirement without a partner for love and even without a partner to share life.*

Gina, a young woman of 70, said to me when I first met her, "I'm depressed and don't have the slightest idea what to do with my life. I thought after my divorce, over ten years ago, that I'd go out and find a nice man and fall in love again and live happily ever after."

She frowned as she continued, "I'm not a Pollyanna type. I know that life is no fairytale, but I felt I could offer a man love and caring. Even though I've had a number of brief affairs I've never found someone to fall in love with. And none of the men fell in love with me. To this day I don't understand that.

"I'm attractive, financially independent, easy to be with, like all sorts of things, including sports and I'm no wallflower. I really put myself out there and find ways to meet many men. I've tried dating services online and connected with a number of men to no avail. Doctor, is something wrong with me? Do I have to be satisfied with my life without love? If that's so, please tell me, and I'll find a way to adjust to life without it."

Donna, another young women of 58, lamented, "I've been on my own for over seven years and zilch, not a man in my life. I've got loads of girlfriends and some men friends, but no lovers. What's the world coming to? Do all the good men hide away or have they given up on women? It hardly pays anymore to even think about it, but a little love and some good sex would certainly be nice."

And finally, Thomas, a mere 76 years of age, chimed in, "You'd think that we men would have it easy. Sure I've dated a lot, but frankly it isn't easy to find the woman of my dreams. Yeah, I'm still dreaming that there's a wonder woman out there for me. But I've had enough. It's just too much trouble to date anymore. I'd rather sit home watching a movie or go out with my buddies or see my grandchildren. But a nice woman would certainly be a treat."

What do these three people have in common? All seek a lover and mate. All appear open to a loving and intimate relationship. And all have apparently given up trying, at least with anything resembling enthusiasm.

Gina admitted that for over five years she'd made no serious attempt to try new venues and activities to meet men, except for periodic forays into Internet dating. Also she decided that it was not worthwhile trying to have male friends, when she enjoys being with her women friends so much.

Donna said that she exhausted the various ways to meet men and decided that the dating game was too hard and unrewarding. "So why bother," were her words.

And Thomas prefers to be alone rather than face the frustration of seeking ways to meet women. He had tried five or six dating services over a period of several unrewarding years. He tried senior citizen activities and church programs. He sought new friends in college and extension division classes. He walked with the Sierra Club and went to a couple of Valentine Day dances. There were no sparks set off in any of these activities. So he stopped attending them and reluctantly stopped searching for other avenues to meet someone.

Are these three people typical of the older single population? I'm not certain, but I do know that there are millions just like them. They want to meet new friends and find that wonderful person who will become an intimate and loving partner. They're attractive, young at heart, vital people, who had once been in love and still are very capable of giving and receiving love. Even those who had developed doubts about their lovability and shy away from contacts are inwardly interested in finding love and sharing life with a partner.

What else might be behind the lack of motivation and persistence to seek out new intimate partners? Since most single older people have been married and either divorced or widowed, their pasts can't be ignored as they enter the single world again. Many have become cautious based on previous experiences. They have gone through one or more marriages where conflicts with a spouse have made them wary of forming another lifetime relationship.

Deliberate and very conscious efforts must be made to overcome this residual doubt and wariness. The future does not have to repeat the past, even if it was bleak and unhappy. You will find ways to meet people who desire closeness and intimacy and want to make a new relationship work. This is no time to deliberately avoid seeking a new partner.

Most important is realizing that the search itself will lead to many new adventures and friends. No one can predict whether anyone will meet a person with whom a permanent attachment is made. There is no doubt, however, that with the right frame of mind the search itself will be rewarding and fulfilling. There are many avenues that await you as you open the door to new ventures and experiences.

STARTING THE SEARCH

Where do you start to look? Some might react and say that they've tried everything. Perhaps you did, but it's no reason to assume that beyond the "everything" there is nothing more. Let's start our search by accessing Google. Under the heading of "retirement books," Google lists countless references. As with most Google references their lead books are usually helpful and might provide avenues for new activities and directions.

Next you might want to access Amazon.com where you'll find a listing of most books on retirement currently available. As with Google the books that Amazon places at the head of their lists are not only their most popular books in the field, but are often books worth reading. Part of your search lies in seeking books that attract you. You're looking for books that point out new avenues for exploration. New friends await you in these endeavors. Keep in mind that many of the books on retirement focus on financial security. I have deliberately excluded that essential area from my book since it is so adequately covered by other books, brokerage houses, educational courses and common sense.

After regaling yourself with Google's and Amazon's efforts to assist you, it's time to venture out of your home to the library. Browsing among their books on retirement should give you a number of clues to guide you to a variety of activities. As you make notes and photocopy ideas from their books, as well as borrowing a few, you're taking steps forward.
There is no doubt that you will discover many things previously unknown to you.

So now that you know that there are virtually unlimited books and paths to seek and search, it's more a matter of your dedication to forge new directions. By keeping in mind that everything you try is for your own edification you will not necessarily be disappointed when you do not meet a potential partner. However, you will most certainly meet new friends, have fun and add much spice to your life. That in itself is a good reason to take some of these paths.

So join me as we move out into the world and seek actual activities. They are often a direct path to new friends and to love. Consider this a **partial list**, which may include some you have already tried:

- Extension division classes at high schools and colleges.
- Private education programs, such as *The Learning Annex.*
- Senior citizen clubs and activities, often set up by your city.
- Church and synagogue senior groups.
- Charities of any sort. Many people enjoy those involved with social events tied to aiding health groups, cancer research, children's needs, hospitals, and animal shelters.
- Environmental organizations often welcome members to participate in activities directed to saving our natural resources, as well as fighting pollution and global warming. Many people find much satisfaction participating in one or more environmental organizations.

- In particular, the Sierra Club offers numerous outings for those of you who enjoy hiking, camping, biking and exploring. There are Sierra groups for all ages, both married and single. You are bound to find similarly spirited friends among them. Besides you will trek in the most beautiful outdoor areas in your part of the state.
- The Environmental Alliance for Senior Involvement (EASI) is another excellent organization to stimulate seniors to actively participate in many important environmental programs. If you want to find out how to better our world, EASI may be for you.
- Opportunities to volunteer in a number of organizations directed toward helping others are readily available. For those who would like to combine their search with travel, Action Without Borders can assist you. They list thousands of resources, nationally and internationally, and can help guide you.
- AARP is another good resource for these organizations.

INTERNET DATING

So far, I have not specifically suggested organizations and groups that necessarily lead you to finding a partner, although many indirectly will do that. A direct link to meeting potential partners is Internet dating services, which have memberships in the millions. There are literally hundreds of different dating services that allow you to select those that best fit your expectations and agenda. Since individuals are separated by age, you can focus on the age group that attracts you.

If you view Internet dating as an adventure without high expectations you will, at the very least, have fun and meet some interesting people.   As in most other circumstances it is still a numbers game to meet that special person. But unless you play the numbers your chances dwindle rather sharply. Internet dating offers you a large and varied group of potential dates, friends and lovers.

In recent years Internet dating has become more prominent among the older population. Seniors no longer frown on using services that put them in touch with other older singles. For many it has become their only resource to meet people for possible romance. Email communication fills time for lonely seniors. Many develop close and even intimate friendships with people they never physically meet. Others prefer to communicate with seniors who live nearby offering the potential of meeting in person.

The general rules of arranging a meeting with an unknown person are now fairly well established. They are similar for all age groups, including older adults. After perusing the profiles of potential new friends, the seeker sends emails to all appealing individuals. They can be of any length but essentially indicate the pleasure in reading their profiles and the desire to know them better. If the recipients like the letter and feel there is compatibility and interest after reading the profile of the sender they reciprocate and correspond. Depending on the number of letters you send out, your inbox may be inundated with responses. Also, of course, you will receive emails initiated by unknown persons. The game of fun and romance has begun.

SAMPLES OF INITIAL EMAIL LETTERS

Dear Mary,
Reading the fascinating description of your gardening experiences resulting in prize roses and dahlias sounded so much like something that I would do that it was a foregone conclusion that I would write to you. Not only do I love flowers but your interest in travel and music also resonated with me.

I have also been married and divorced, which you will no doubt notice if you are inclined to read my profile, which I hope you will. Although I don't have a pet at the moment I love dogs and can easily imagine having fun with your retriever. I would certainly never feel your dog was a problem as you indicated that some men do.

Although we don't live right around the corner from each other, we're definitely within driving distance. I understand that long distance relationships are not for you.

I would love to hear from you.

Warmly,

Comments

This letter specifically alludes to several activities mentioned in the profile. Since many people email each other after only looking at the photos many women are hesitant to respond to letters that don't indicate that their profiles were read.

It also indicates a shared interest in a special hobby.

It makes clear that that the writer loves dogs and her dog would be welcomed.

No mention is made of the photo(s) in the profile since it is apparent that a person would not attempt to respond to a profile without feeling some attraction to the photo. Also, it has become fairly well known that many photographs do not adequately represent the person. Nevertheless, photos do stimulate many emails responses in Internet dating and should be appealing.

SAMPLE NO. 2

Dear John,

I've been reading dating profiles for several years but yours is the first that mentioned that your interest in travel has made you into a bona fide explorer of Los Angeles. I was really surprised to hear about some of your discoveries in Griffith Park that I had never known about. And I thought I knew LA.

I love that you spend time tutoring young children in math and offer your time to young children's athletic teams. It must be fun being an assistant coach for Little League teams. It's obvious that you love children. I imagine that your own grandchildren must have a wonderful grandfather.

I couldn't help but notice that one of your photographs was a picture taken at Yosemite, an all-time favorite vacation spot that I have visited many times. It was actually a wonderful shot of Half Dome in the background apparently taken near dusk, if I read the shadows right.

I hope that you read my profile and feel inclined to write me. It would be fun sharing some ideas about LA since you may have realized that I also love to wander around the city. I also enjoy exploring the Santa Monica Mountains, since I love to hike.

Regards,

Comments

Your profile touched this woman as she obviously resonated with elements of your interests and lifestyle. There is little purpose in responding to a profile where there's not a good chance of finding compatibility in at least one important area of your life. Also, this indicates why it is important to include such interests when you write your profile.

Her reaction to your photo was the nature of the picture and the artistry involved. It's obvious she looked closely at your pictures and just didn't react to your appearance.

Your interest as a retiree in helping young children also appealed to her. This reveals or demonstrates that she, in turn, also loves young children and would support and even share your interests.

SAMPLE NO. 3

Dear Carol,

In a nutshell, I thought your profile and picture and the feelings that came from them fit exactly into what I'd like to read and feel when I check out a profile. And that's what I hope will happen when you read mine. We have so much in common; at least from my view of our profiles, that I felt that writing to you was imperative. So here's my letter and I hope that you write back.

We could have fun comparing restaurants when we write and maybe later talk since you're apparently a lover of ethnic food and I assume a gourmet cook. Have you ever eaten at Dante's a delightful Italian restaurant in Santa Monica? Makes you feel like you're in Tuscany.

Hoping to hear from you,

Comments

This letter though brief is personal and enthusiastic and ends with acknowledging one area in which they apparently share an interest.

Sometimes the emotion in the initial email is the stimulus that causes a recipient to respond. Two people who have never met are leery of connecting without a definite stimulus or potential link. The Internet is no longer new. Most older people have tried it and many have been dating that way for years. Many have become discouraged due to the lack of finding more permanent connections. Therefore, in your emails always find a way of expressing a meaningful sentiment, putting in humor, noting common interests. Above all your correspondence needs to be very positive.

SAMPLE NO. 4

Dear Dan,

I loved your profile and picture and although my letter is very brief it comes from my careful reading of your profile. My son also graduated from San Diego State where you obtained your Masters. It wasn't clear whether you're still teaching high school but it's worth noting that I also work part time to keep busy.

Please take a look at my profile and with a big smile write.

Best wishes,

Comments

Very brief yet deliberately made personal. Most people today will just delete anything which seems routine or a form letter. You need to write in a way that at the very least the recipient checks on your profile, and then it's in the hands of fate. Your profile should reveal your personal interests, written with feeling and some style. You need to express likes and dislikes that are truly pertinent to who you are. No point in hiding things that are essential to establish a meaningful relationship. By the time you have become a senior there is no need to waste time or write in a way that either gets no responses or overloads you with responses based on made up material.

Honest, sensitive and personal profiles tend to garner responses. Your detailed information will hopefully stimulate responses from compatible individuals. Whether you're looking for a date, a friend, a lover or eventually marriage you need to start out with connecting.

EMAIL AND TELEPHONE

From this time forward many avenues open. **Email communication** can go on for a lengthy period or the two persons may decide to talk on the **telephone** almost immediately. Some people bypass this phase and after the email has established the connection they arrange to meet. However, I personally believe that telephone communication is useful as a next step for better assessing each other. If both are comfortable with the interchange they can arrange to meet.

FIRST MEETING

This meeting is generally for coffee, tea or a drink and often takes place in the early afternoon. If two people strike a responsive note, the meeting could be extended. Otherwise, such interchanges tend to be brief. Most people can assess within a half hour if the potential for a friendship or romance is slight.

Many people enjoy the brief contact and share certain intimacies even when it is clear that they will not meet again. On the other hand, many of these brief coffee dates may go on for hours, when two people find a camaraderie and connection that draw them together.

These meetings can be difficult for those who hate the idea of being evaluated and tested. Both persons are usually somewhat nervous despite knowing the odds are not high for making a real connection. But this is not different from other meetings with an unknown person or a blind date set up before the Internet was established. Such meetings were just as difficult.

Naturally if the meeting is pleasant and has aroused curiosity, at the very least, or better, a strong attraction or "chemistry", then they will most likely arrange to meet again, usually for lunch or dinner. Yes, "chemistry" happens at all ages and with just as much excitement and anticipation for the future.

Other ways to meet for the initial mutual interview are to meet in a park or at the beach for a walk. If the walk is pleasing to both, then coffee can follow. Some people arrange to meet in a local museum and even to attend a concert. There are no rules that determine when and how this first meeting takes place but caution should dictate safety since the person is unknown. Judgment, intuition, and openness play a part as meetings are set up.

CONNECTING THROUGH TRAVEL

Another venue to meet friends and even potential partners is by traveling. If adventure is in your blood and travel beckons, then by all means do it. However, in the interest of meeting other seniors, consider taking trips where single elders go. Elderhostel is an organization that now has nearly 8,000 courses and travels to over 90 countries. Many single older adults attend these courses and sometimes lifelong friends are made.

Many travel organizations arrange tours for single travelers paying a single supplement and joining the larger group. Some set up tours where singles are the only or the predominant group. Either way don't hesitate to travel when alone. Travelers tend to be friendly and you can quickly find companionship and possibly friendship traveling with tour groups.

There are several tour organizations that can help you find a travel mate of the same or opposite sex, if desired. Many older people have found Seniorsmatch.com to be helpful in arranging for compatible travel companions. This is less for romance than companionship and gives you the option of not traveling alone if other companions are not available. The usual cautions are obvious in making such arrangements.

Many other senior activities offer stimulation, fulfillment and purpose in your life without necessarily helping you find love. Nevertheless, the more activities you undertake or participate in the more likely someone will appear that strikes that special note. Not only from direct meetings but from new friends who like you and want to introduce you to a "special" person.

There are many people, just like you, eager to find someone to share life with and who are waiting to meet you. Many have become discouraged and only need an introduction or new impetus to reengage in reaching out. You're starting on a new quest that will provide you with a new exciting life. And no doubt love is somewhere out there for you.

REACHING OUT

However, having a happy and satisfying relationship in your older age is not dependent on having a love relationship. It is more dependent on a willingness to reach out to others and a readiness to accept new friends. From these new friends you're more apt to find that special person you seek. At the very least, you will have a more bountiful and meaningful life sharing yourself with others. And you may find that love now comes in various forms.

Love is present in many other guises and often deeply binds two people in a wonderful and fulfilling relationship. Perhaps above all, we wish to experience that elusive "love at first sight" where there are no boundaries and often little reality. Such feelings are little different from their occurrence in adolescence. Although such transcendent moments do occur in love relationships, true love is apt to develop more slowly from friendship and shared experiences.

The mutual caring and nurturing of good friends can lead to a special and highly responsive relationship without sharing sex that ultimately leads to love. The love evolves from mutual respect, trust and intimacy. Such love can touch the souls of two people who share deeply.

Sometimes sex is part of this kind of caring relationship and adds another element to it. At times the sex can even be a powerful and exciting component of what started as a deeply nurturing relationship. Perhaps ideally we would enjoy finding a new friend where a feeling of intimacy and caring evolves and leads to the heightened pleasure of sex. Some people may have several such caring relationships without sex being part of them.

Sharing sex with someone you love is different and generally more fulfilling than casual sex. A heightened degree of excitement depends on many factors and certainly can take place with a relative stranger. However, an older couple in love brings experience, caring and makes a concerted effort to attain mutual satisfaction. As long as sex is mutually desired it can become an important and frequent component of a love relationship.

Eugene, a 76 years old man, lost his wife after 45 years of a happy and fulfilling marriage. For two years he pined and dreamed of his former life that had abruptly ended. Each day he recalled the tenderness in his wife's touch and the caresses they shared. In his mind only Louise could exist. No other woman could ever take her place.

Louise had developed acute leukemia and had died within two weeks of the diagnosis. Eugene was devastated and despite the encouragement of his two children and friends he refused to see other women. He remained depressed and withdrawn, spending his time reading and listening to music, almost always alone. Only the devotion of several male friends induced him to leave the house for short walks and an occasional movie and dinner.

Finally, his wife's younger sister, Clara, bolstered by their close relationship, persuaded him to attend a small dinner party given to honor the publication of a book by a close friend. At the party, Clara had arranged for Eugene to meet, Natalie, an attractive and sensitive woman. During the evening they became friendly and Natalie drew from him the anguish and hopelessness he had felt after his wife had died. Before the evening ended he had accepted an invitation from her to a small dinner.

A warm, perceptive and outgoing woman, Diana, a widow of five years, had been invited by Natalie to the same dinner. Diana had been told of Eugene's difficulty in breaking free of his love for his wife. She knew that a man's preoccupation and obsession with his previous marriage would be a difficult hurdle to overcome, even if they hit it off. However, she also knew that a man who had had a long and loving marriage was more apt to be a kind and loving man to another woman. Whether he could finally put his love for his deceased wife to rest remained to be seen. She had lost her husband to cancer five years earlier and had longed to rekindle her love and intimacy with a special man.

Eugene and Diana connected that evening and began to date. Although they shared many interests her outgoing nature initially caused some consternation since she wanted him to join her activities and he was still unable to face the pressures of a new social life. At times it appeared that the barriers were insurmountable and little would come from their developing friendship.

Typical angry scenes erupted. "Eugene, it will do you good to attend the concert. You love music and you once enjoyed going to the music hall."

Eugene's response was always, "Diana, I'm not interested in spending time driving downtown and being in that crowd. I enjoy listening on my stereo."

"It's not the same."

"To me it's better."

"You're so stubborn."

"Diana, maybe we should go our own ways. We have too many arguments."

"What do you mean? We have very few arguments."

"All right I grant you that. It's because you don't always try to pressure me to go out."

"Eugene, it's not healthy staying home all the time."

"I'm not home all the time."

"You're exasperating."

"Just go to the concert yourself and leave me alone."

These kinds of interaction occurred at times as their relationship continued and became complicated by children, grandchildren, lifestyles, interests, time with friends, health matters and the desire for sex which eventually came into the foreground.

In recent years Eugene had difficulty in having erections and was hesitant to approach her sexually. He could enjoy sex but only in certain ways where intercourse was not included. Although his wife never found their sex life wanting he knew that her love over decades made their romantic life able to adjust to any kind of sex.

Several months went by before Diana decided to broach the subject. She had already assumed that he had trouble with sex since he was otherwise affectionate and seemed to desire close and affectionate contact. However, he refused to go to bed with her saying that he wasn't quite ready.

After discussing his sexual problems in his counseling with me I convinced him that most women are completely understanding of erection problems in men, which occur for many reasons as men get older. For many men Viagra helps overcome the dysfunction. I suggested that he tell Diana of his problem and fears and his wish to try Viagra. I also indicated that if Viagra didn't work and there was any difficulty in enjoying intercourse then manual and oral sex that he had enjoyed with his wife was usually acceptable to understanding women. Also a few sessions of sex therapy, accompanied by Diana, would conceivably help him overcome his erectile disorder.

Eugene finally approached Diana and explained his sex problem. She laughed and said to her sex was involved with intimacy, closeness and their growing love. It tuned out that though Viagra helped it wasn't essential for having sex. Diana was quite content with sex without intercourse and they quickly found genuine sexual compatibility.

A short time later Eugene had overcome his depression and any tendency toward withdrawal. His relationship with Diana was definitely on the upswing and they were planning a long vacation trip. They looked forward to an exciting and loving relationship. He ended his counseling ready to live the "good life" as he called it.

The story of Eugene and Diana is heartwarming, yet typical. Two people, one withdrawn and isolated, the other outgoing and participating in much of life, found each other through the intercession of family and friends who refused to see either linger in a non-loving lifestyle.

Whether friends are needed to help or not, it behooves all seniors who live alone and desire to establish an intimate and long term relationship to use whatever resources are necessary to facilitate their quest. They should not lose hope as they continue to search until that special person is found. Even if not, as I've already indicated, new friends and new activities will certainly help fulfill one's retirement life.

THE VICISSITUDES OF LOVE

> *Love is often expressed through tenderness and warmth. You relate differently than with others. You feel more protective, more apt to want to share thoughts and ideas. You are more playful and childlike and spontaneously burst into song and dance. You want to play more, especially when the two of you are alone. The desire for quick weekend holidays and extensive travel is ever-present. You tend to have secret hideaways and special interests unknown to others. In a sense two lovers share a private world.*

Sharing inner and personal thoughts with an empathic and understanding person should alert you to the possibility that you are experiencing love. For many people merely touching that special person awakens a feeling of closeness and intimacy. As you may realize, love is a many faceted emotion and appears in many forms. You want to experience as many as possible.

Love as fantasy awakens excitement and the imagination. As we daydream of love that remains to be discovered, we enjoy vicarious pleasures of what might be. Such day dreaming can often be a prelude to what may develop in real life and becomes an inducement to seek out relationships. However, for some individuals, fantasies may become highly satisfying in themselves but should not impede attempts to meet real people.

Lorraine, 62 years old, came to see me because of depression, compulsive eating and loneliness. She spent a part of each day writing down the fantasies of her secret love life. She had become so immersed in fantasizing that she was reluctant to break the pattern by actually seeking a real-life partner. "I feel wonderful when I imagine being made love to by the handsomest and cleverest man alive," she exclaimed. "No book can top my sexual experiences. Everyday I write a new story. Why should I look elsewhere? With myself I'm guaranteed satisfaction. And I don't always need to have an orgasm every time I imagine being loved."

In her search for love Lorraine had created stories about losing weight, joining a fitness center, looking great in attractive and appealing clothes, participating in a hiking club and meeting people on bicycle trips. Many of her stories involved interests and activities that were not sexual and a few evolved out of a desire to become spiritual.

In her effort to turn her life around, Lorraine decided to follow some of her stories. She was somewhat overweight and started to diet. Shortly later she joined a fitness center and became a serious exerciser. Later she added Yoga to her exercise routine. She quickly separated her real attempts from her fantasies and began to make her life vital and meaningful.

She loved nature and joined several nature groups and for the first time in her life developed a true interest in hiking and bicycling. With the Sierra Club she began to explore the Santa Monica Mountains and made new friendships with several women.

Within eight months she had become a totally different woman. She had lost 30 pounds and was now at her ideal weight of 125 pounds. She hiked many local mountains and rode her bike several days each week. She went on walking tours of England and France where she met a number of active and vigorous older people, many in retirement. During her "first-century" bike ride she met her dream man. He was 71. As far as I know they are still together.

By changing from a passive person using fantasies for pleasure, Lorraine had become actively involved in changing her life. Her stories were now seen as preludes to her new and very real life.

REFLECTIONS

Is there a bona fide formula for finding that desired love relationship? The answer is YES.

"Yes," means maintaining the motivation and persistence to find venues to meet people plus "keeping your eyes open." Many opportunities exist to reach out to an attractive person. One of them could become a friend and even a lover. Don't think that being older stops anyone from flirting, offering a friendly hello and attempting to strike up a conversation. Don't allow your being older to interfere with the youthful attitude of making connections with people, including potential lovers.

Love can develop when two people deeply share certain interests and activities. This can also be the basis for good and lasting friendships. These activities can include art, music, nature, walks, movies, sports, special dinners, travel, religion and spirituality. Any of these areas can bring two people together and become the impetus for a love relationship to grow. Whether we find new love relationships or share love with special friends or love the activities that enliven our lives, it is love that is the magical balm that vitalizes our existence.

As the desire for a more spiritual existence evolves, another way to meet new friends develops. Exploring and cultivating spirituality with someone of like mind is a wonderful way to bring two people closer. Participating in spiritual events as part of the continuing search for spiritual attainment can be an especially important part of growing intimacy. At times such a search can bring a couple into a better understanding of their religious beliefs and add another ingredient to their expanding relationship.

When a new friendship is formed, find all possible ways to enliven it. If it ends, look back on it as a time of temporary or transient pleasure and go on. Too frequently, seniors tend to stop reaching out and erect a wall to ward off potential relationships. Such walls often keep out the people who might offer friendship and love. Aim to expand your horizons and remain open to new friends and activities. The treasure is found by those who continue to search. And who knows in what form or manner such treasures exist.

CONCLUSIONS

Love is boundless and beckons to us. We need to reach out and grasp it. By developing a positive mental state your journey will be successful. The sources exist. Activities are plentiful. From the Internet to travel, to educational programs, to sports, to creative pursuits and environmental programs the list is endless. The quest for love awakens the imagination and revitalizes us. And what a way to grow young in retirement.

Chapter Three

BARRIERS TO LOVE

Not knowing when the dawn will come, I open every door.

—Emily Dickinson

A true conception of the relation between the sexes will not admit of conqueror and conquered; it knows but of one great thing; to give of one's self boundlessly, in order to find one's self richer, deeper, better.

—Emma Goldman

Do you believe you are loveless? Are you unable to love?

You may find you are without love in your life due to divorce, loss, never having been married or difficulty in finding a partner. With time on your hands you can now seek new friends and a new love relationship. But what if you believe that you're loveless because of an inability to love? You feel that you are doomed to be alone and have given up looking. That negativism needs to end. Everyone can find love and I'm going to show you many ways, avenues and techniques to seek and find that love. If you believe that you are unable to love and this doubt has grown so it is now difficult to pursue love, then take heart;

you are about to set out on a new path to find the love you seek.

Is it possible that some of us are truly unable to love? I doubt it. I doubt that anyone who desires love is incapable of overcoming that inner barrier that has forestalled the search and discovery of love. In this chapter I'll describe how to overcome the barriers to love and reveal ways that all people can love more deeply and even find love where it had not existed. Sometimes it is not until a person faces retirement that the emptiness of a loveless life becomes a crucial issue to overcome.

Elizabeth, a tall and strikingly beautiful woman, preparing to retire, came to see me to help her overcome a loveless life. Her first words described the serious dilemma she faced. "Doctor, I'm depressed and feel hopeless. I'm 64 years old and have never been in love. I don't even know if I can love. I go through the motions of showing affection and pretending how happy I am, but it's all pretense. I don't want to live this way."

Such was the introduction to another of the love-lonely people who face their senior years fearful of isolation and aloneness. Elizabeth fit the pattern of those who avoid the issue altogether. While in the work force or being married such beliefs tend to be hidden. But when facing the new world of retirement a vision of emptiness coupled with fears that go with this part of the life cycle envelop them.

Elizabeth, unmarried, epitomized this quandary. After retiring from her work as a buyer for a large antique chain she spent considerable time reading, attending classes at the university and spending time with friends. During these early months of retirement her "handicap" in being unable to love really hit her. She no longer traveled nor met stimulating people, who had helped her ignore her problem.

Traveling to foreign cities and being single had given her access to many men, who had always been attracted to her. She kept busy and ignored the signs of being unable to love. She had affairs with good men and a few not so good. But it was always the same. The men frequently said they loved her and were excited by her. However, she felt nothing or very little. She had become expert in pretending to like them, but had never told any man that she loved him.

When each affair ended a new one started. She believed that it was only a matter of time before the right man would come along and she'd fall in love. But it never happened. She slowly recognized that not only hadn't she fallen in love but all her feelings were feigned. She had lived as though she were a loving woman but deep down she had developed barriers to loving. She enjoyed sex, which masqueraded as love and closeness. She imagined that she was loving back. For years she hid the truth from herself.

Accepting her handicap was not easy but now opened the possibility of truly overcoming the barriers that prevented her from finding love. I gave her the needed reassurance that age was no impediment to finding love. Being able to love is inherent in people of all ages.

I thought of the many patients I have seen over the years who have expressed similar feelings. For those who can love openly and easily it is difficult to fathom the desperation and inner emptiness of people like Elizabeth. Many spend a lifetime pretending and eventually coming to accept that they can't love or inwardly believe that what they feel is love.

> *The need to believe in one's lovability is a powerful force tied to self-esteem and a sense of well-being. Only by believing that we can love and are lovable can we believe in our deeper self-value. Such beliefs are often tied to a feeling of spirituality and a sense of one's essential goodness. Experiencing love becomes necessary to stimulate and heighten self-esteem.*

Not being able to find a person to love may be tied to shyness, passivity, not knowing where or how to seek lovers or harboring a deep belief of being unlovable. This latter belief had induced Elizabeth to enter therapy and influences many people to avoid making connections with potential lovers.

Most people find it extremely unpleasant to imagine that they are unlovable or perhaps even worse, that some deep inner feeling is preventing them from finding lovers. They, therefore, continue to seek love hoping that they will finally find that elusive person to love and to love them. Over time they realize that persons they are attracted to avoid them or only engage in brief relationships. Their incompatibility quickly becomes clear. Other lonely people are frequently desired by potential partners but time after time they put up impenetrable barriers and reject them.

A common element frequently exists in many adults who either become attracted to unavailable or incompatible people or who reject worthy suitors or lovers who seek them out. Unwittingly, they are struggling with an inner belief of being unlovable and that something is wrong with them. They, therefore, back away from potential lovers not wanting anyone to get close and really see who they are inside.

Both groups of people actually fear real intimacy and closeness and erect powerful defenses against recognizing these fears. They find deficiencies and defects with their potential mates and begin to believe that there is no one who can measure up to their need to be loved. They justify their attitude by finding fault with those who come too close.

Reactions to rejection can follow several scenarios. First, there may be a strong sense of loss and worthlessness on being rejected. One may not recognize that a part of them engineered the rejection due to an inner sense of worthlessness.

Another possible outcome develops out of the conviction that the lover was not as worthy as first considered. In a sense their being rejected is converted into their degrading the initially idealized lover. This provides another defense against an inner sense of unworthiness.

The second group who constantly reject potential mates finds fault in all those who are attracted to them. By rejecting these people first they avoid believing that the problem is in them. Eventually they believe there is no one who exists that they could ever love. They finally accept being alone without love.

The belief in one's capacity to love and to feel loved can fluctuate. Some people feel they can love certain individuals and only when stress intervenes do they have doubts. For others a deep emptiness occurs periodically appearing without warning and seemingly without provocation. Only by careful evaluation can the causes of such periodic reactions be determined. Frequently it occurs from minor slights, often ignored, that prey on inner doubts until they erupt in depression and self-doubt. For some the dread of never feeling love is constant, much as it was with Elizabeth.

Fortunately, there are many who can take in love in varying degrees and thus have a greater sense of self and much less desperation. They are usually those who love selected people, such as their children or parents. Even so, they too suffer from pangs of doubt and frequently succumb to a deep sense of emptiness.

MENTAL IMAGERY

For those who have **doubts about their lovability or self-value** I would like to introduce the first of a group of **Mental Imagery** exercises that can facilitate overcoming these specific negative thoughts. The use of Mental Imagery is now widespread and goes far beyond its use by professional athletes. Artists, writers, actors, inventors and those expanding their creativity and imagination utilize its principles. I have used it successfully in my clinical practice to help patients overcome a variety of emotional problems and develop a more positive attitude about life. I will use these principles for a number of effective exercises throughout this book. I suggest that you read the **addendum** at the end of the book and get an idea of what Mental Imagery is and how it is used to change mindsets.

Imagery exercises work best when practiced in a state of deep relaxation or an alpha state, the state of increased auto-suggestibility. Please review Exercise No. 4 on page 28 for information about the alpha state.

Although any relaxation technique will suffice, I have found that a very simple method that I call the **Rag Doll** facilitates your entering a state of deep relaxation (alpha state) in 7 or 8 seconds.

EXERCISE NO. 5: THE RAG DOLL TECHNIQUE

> Sit in a comfortable chair. Relax your body. Close your eyes. Visualize yourself as a rag doll. To enhance this visual picture it may help to shake your arms and legs a few moments in a loose manner like a rag doll.
>
> Take a slow, deep breath. Hold a few seconds. Then as you slowly exhale, imagine pouring your mental self into your rag doll self. Take another slow, deep breath and again slowly exhale and once more pour your mental self into your rag doll self. You are now in a deep state of relaxation.

Practice the rag doll technique a few times until you are comfortable with it, and can truly feel the deep relaxation that is conducive to practicing the imagery exercises.

For those who desire to gauge the timing of your breathing, count to four on inhaling, hold your breath to the count of two and then exhale to the count of four. As soon as you feel comfortable with the rate of your breathing, there is no need to count. After a brief period of use most people only take one deep breath to induce the alpha state.

Setting up a simple **Mental Imagery** exercise is easy. You first determine the **Imagery setting**, which is the feeling or behavior that you want to correct or change (the negative mindset). You immediately follow with the imagery that will destroy or **eradicate** the negative belief. You end with an **affirmation** that repeats and solidifies your new belief. Simple, but effective, when repeated over a period of time.

As your imagery setting you can use any belief you wish but for the sake of demonstrating how the exercise is set up

I'll use a deep feeling of laziness as the negative mindset, which occurs at times in many of us. However, you can imagine whatever symptoms, attitudes or behavior that you have that in your mind disparage you or in some way make you believe you're unacceptable to yourself and/or the opposite sex. These are negative mindsets.

EXERCISE NO. 6: CHANGING NEGATIVE MINDSETS

> Go into a state of relaxation using the rag doll technique. Imagine feeling that you are the laziest person alive and it's just too hard to make the effort to get up and be more active. You are shriveled up on a sofa or lying in bed or passively glued to the TV. Exaggerate how you look and feel. Suddenly, as though struck by a magical light you stand up, raise your hands high and exclaim that you no longer feel lazy or empty, that you will never again feel negative toward yourself. Say to yourself with conviction, "I am a good, wise and vital person. I will live with a feeling of love and joy and nothing will stand in my way to accomplish whatever I wish."

Perhaps by now, if you have used the first few exercises I described, you have become aware of your inner doubts or negative mindsets. If not, allow your feelings to surface. No one is free of some doubts or feelings of inferiority. If there are many such symptoms you may prefer to break this exercise into several parts but there is no harm in lumping them into one composite negative mindset.

Name or briefly describe what you feel and intensify your reactions. The stronger your feelings the more effective are the gradual changes in your beliefs. For example, you might say, "I feel unintelligent and ugly. I'm too short or too tall. I'm too fat or too thin. I'm easily aroused to anger and am overly critical with others. I judge people harshly and find faults with everyone. I feel inferior to others although I think I'm really superior." These are a few of the emotions that make people suffer and feel unlovable.

Once you have established in your mind the negative things you want to change you say them with deep conviction and complete belief. If you can't yet believe in this mental technique, imagine its power until you can finally accept it. These exercises are effective only if you believe in the power of the mind to change you. You can believe them because they work over time.

An Example of a Complete Exercise

After entering a state of deep relaxation you state the belief you want to change. "I feel stupid and ugly." The antidote immediately occurs. A brilliant light flashes in your mind and your thoughts become extremely positive. You know you are intelligent and beautiful. You end with an affirmation. "I'll never again feel unworthy or negative in any way. I am an intelligent, beautiful and loving person."

Since negative mindsets influence all of us and we want to rid our minds of this kind of thinking, I suggest that you use an end-state imagery exercise to accompany Exercise No. 6. End-state imagery is set up to show how you will appear after you have completely overcome the negative mindset you are seeking to change. Remember the best Mental Imagery is developed by the individual so that it fits him and serves his needs. Be imaginative and free. Imagery works and you have nothing to lose by trying it. Believe in its power. In a way this is akin to believing in your ability to change.

You are still in the relaxed state so there is no need to again induce relaxation. You now have two exercises that are done sequentially in a single exercise period.

EXERCISE NO. 7: LIFE AS A LOVING AND LOVED PERSON
(End-state imagery)

See yourself in a situation where you are obviously loved. Walk into a crowd of people who immediately reach out to you and exclaim how wonderful it is to see you. Leave and begin to walk in a park where you meet a person who obviously loves you as you acknowledge your own love. Embrace each other for the amazing people you are. You and your lover are lying in bed feeling exhilarated knowing you have enjoyed incredible love making.

End-state imagery can be used whenever you decide on making some change in your behavior or mindsets. Many use it as a form of affirmation independent of any desire to change. To them it starts the day on a positive note or sets the mood when they sit down to write, paint or create a gourmet meal. Remember, end-state imagery is always very positive and shows you in the very best light. It's "good-feeling" imagery.

THE MENTAL IMAGERY EXERCISE PROGRAM

Throughout this book I'll introduce many imagery exercises. Select those that work for you. Your objective is to create an exercise package that meets your needs for change. Do them at one sitting in the manner I describe below.

Remember, don't put any time limits or restraints on these exercises. Imagery takes time to work, so don't expect them to suddenly change your attitude or behavior. No matter how long it takes it is essential that you maintain a very positive attitude. One day you will begin to feel different.

Many other activities and influences will be facilitating your changes as well. I'm introducing many techniques for you to try and/or use. You should take what appeals to you. If any of them seems unrealistic, fanciful or unproductive, read on for other ways to make your retirement period better. For now think of yourself as a positive, enthusiastic, creative and adventurous explorer of new ideas for self-change for making your life wholesome and vital.

The Daily Practice of Mental Imagery

Repeat the exercises 5, 20 or more times a day.   Each exercise will only take about 8-10 seconds. All other imagery exercises should be added to the same session, done sequentially. You can complete five or six exercises per session, within approximately 50 seconds plus 8 seconds for the Rag Doll. All the exercises are done during the same period of relaxation. Once you go into this state you can do whatever exercises fit your particular needs. By repeating a group of six exercises ten times a day you are only using ten minutes of time spread over a full day. It will be well worth the time.

SELF-LOVE

To overcome the belief you are not lovable you need to begin the process of reversing this idea. You need to accept that you are a lovable person. Love yourself for the wonderful person you are. In other words the true antidote you seek is SELF-LOVE. In the final analysis the question is, "Do you love yourself?"

What is self-love? Self-love has been bandied around so much we sometimes think it only means selfishness or over-involvement with personal needs. That is one form of self-love, sometimes called narcissism, ego-centrism or self-absorption. However, what I'm speaking about is the kind of self-love that is similar to what a person feels who is loved by another. Only in this case you love yourself. Instead of being selfish it is a feeling of inner fullness. Such fullness gives rise to an abundance of positive feelings toward others that comes from a strong belief of one's inner worth. Such people tend to be bountiful and very giving. They are empathic and capable of connecting to others and giving love abundantly.

When Elizabeth pondered that meaning of self-love she said, "I know that is something I don't feel. I don't give things easily to anyone. I have trouble giving a gift or helping someone who never gives me anything in return.

Also, I often think of what I will gain by doing something for someone. If I think I won't profit from the relationship, I find all sorts of excuses to avoid doing things with that person."

Elizabeth is not alone in her struggle to be a giving person. Rather than finding fault with yourself when you come to a similar realization and admit this frailty to yourself, use this insight as the first step in making changes. If you give in order to receive you do not feel the inner pleasure of giving love. Also when something is given back by reciprocation it is not necessarily because of abundance but frequently because of social need, guilt, or a wish to be loved or admired.

> *Your goal is to be a loving and giving person. To become that person it is helpful to visualize experiences that fit your new view of yourself. You are commencing to change who you are. You are starting to become who you want to be.*

EXERCISE NO. 8: LOVING OTHERS

Relax using the rag doll or other technique. See yourself in a negative light. Example, I'm the most non-giving and non-loving person alive. I want to be different. Suddenly out of nowhere or from an epiphany in your mind you change into the most giving and loving person. See yourself giving love to others. You can give gifts to children, alms to a person in need, help someone blind cross the street, say something positive to someone who feels down. You will imagine their response as loving and with gratitude. A child can show glee and hug you. All the responses will be of love and not of gifts. You will feel that love is a feeling shared and welcomed.

Your affirmation can be. I feel wonderful being the most loving person I can.

In the above exercise select those qualities and actions that resonate with you. As you become more comfortable with imagery you can change the visualizations whenever you wish. The intent in this exercise is to be an increasingly giving and loving person. Eventually you can see yourself filled with love that envelops others that come in contact with you. Remember this is going on in your mind with the idea of changing who you are. Believe it. You have nothing to lose and everything to gain. If this seems silly and improbable, just move on. This book has many other ideas to make your senior life more rewarding.

For disbelievers I often suggest that to every person they meet in a single day to say hello, smile broadly and comment on the beautiful day and wish them well. You will almost always get a positive response and unless you've set up an impenetrable wall you will react positively to the return of good wishes and the warmth of the responsive smile.

When you do these imagery experiences always believe in your ability to change and in the power of imagery. If necessary, pretend you believe your fantasies and imagery at first until you sense the changes and the newly found pleasure from your new self.

In the future as you become more open and flexible, you will change whatever you desire. This is the time to start imagining a new you in all areas that you wish. Not only will imagery stimulate your personal development but it will enhance the pleasure you achieve during retirement.

THE POWER OF FRIENDSHIP

In your quest for love follow the paths that appeal to you. Finding that special person is in a way a numbers game. You meet many to find just one. With zest and enthusiasm make a concerted effort to find that elusive love partner using all avenues available.

At times rather than keeping your sights on someone to love you can direct your search to seeking friendships rather than love. Friends are much more available since most people cherish developing new friendships, especially as they get older. In the many areas that you seek lovers you will find many compatible people who would make great friends. Such an approach also serves the purpose of diminishing the strong negative belief of being unlovable. Very often a new friendship develops into a love relationship. Keep in mind that many people seeking a love connection immediately discard the relationship when that elusive "chemistry" is not felt. Potential friendships are thus lost.

In general, it is more likely that friendships will develop from attending a variety of activities and organizations, including education classes, which you may join. The sharing of interests, viewpoints, political and religious beliefs, environmental concerns and various forms of entertainment contribute to developing new friendships.

Elizabeth understood that she needed to change her actual thinking about feeling unloved and incapable of loving. She decided not to seek love but rather to date men as friends. Instead of dwelling on her fear of rejection and the belief that there was no one out there to love or be loved by she enjoyed the relationships without attempting to stimulate them to respond to her. She was surprised to recognize that she was less critical or judgmental.

When you realize that your belief in being unlovable and being unable to love is irrational you have already taken the first step toward overcoming your inability to seek out new friends and eventually new lovers. People need and desire friends and many would welcome the opportunity to share common interests and activities with a new friend. Such a change offers the opportunity to reach out for friendship and develop meaningful relationships with men, women and children.

Thus, as expected, Elizabeth began to feel warmer and closer to certain girlfriends. She felt drawn to children who seemed to respond to her. She tried saying hello to everyone she met and was surprised at the positive reactions she received. She was beginning to reach out to the world about her.

Reach out to the world and the world
reaches out to you. Many of us for

various reasons have drifted away from family and old friends and only in our later years do we attempt to find each other again. It is never too late. Barriers can be overcome through desire and effort. Most people hunger for friendship and love.

BECOMING A LOVING PERSON

Now is the time to not falter. You will find love by giving love. Helping others on a one to one basis and becoming involved in various organizations and activities directed toward giving to others will open the door to friendship and love.

With much enthusiasm Elizabeth started what appeared to be a campaign to become a loving person. She joined several hospital groups to help sick children and older people. She read to the blind and joined several environmental groups to work toward stemming the tide of global warming. She joined a charitable group that collected money to fight cancer.

Elizabeth also made peace with her past and so laid the groundwork to loving herself. She learned to forgive those people in her past who had hurt her. She established a new relationship with her siblings and crept into the hearts of her nieces and nephews and their children. Most important was the awareness of a change in herself. She cried when she described how a small child, Tina, just five, her grandniece, insisted on being with her, sitting on her lap, kissing her cheek, hugging her and laughing with her. "I felt so drawn to her and I knew without any doubt that I truly loved her. I didn't have to wipe away troubling thoughts or anything. I just loved her."

Slowly, inexorably, the love that was in her came alive. She offered so much and so freely that people sought her out. New and old friends entered her life and touched her even as she touched them. Elizabeth was becoming the loving and loved person she had sought.

EXERCISE NO. 9: LOVING YOURSELF (End-state imagery)

> Go into a state of deep relaxation.
> Imagine that you are peering into your inner self and can see the evidence of deep love inside you. Perhaps you see a pristine and completely unembellished inner you. You see love in the form of glistening organs and everything that appears healthy and pulsating with vigor. You know that you are looking into your very soul and it is filled with love. You know that you are a loving person and you feel a deep love for yourself.

REFLECTIONS

Is the story of Elizabeth unique? Can people who have lived devoid of love or having put up barriers to love and intimacy regain the closeness that comes with love? The answer is an unequivocal "yes."

In a way Elizabeth represents all of us entering our older years. Those who have conflicts about loving tend to find ways to feel closeness and intimacy with certain people. They hide the inner conflicts about their limited ability to love. But as they get older their restricted love and intimacy no longer suffice and the urge to reach out for greater love develops. Finding that greater love is the search we need to make.

Elizabeth required psychotherapy to assist her to overcome a deep-seated conflict about the fear of closeness and love. However, most of us can surmount many of our inner obstacles through self-understanding alone. When we sense that our loving is false or pretended and we're only going through the motions of intimacy, we need to pause and take stock of our behavior. Change depends on our awareness and acceptance of our individual problems. None of us can overcome anything unless we acknowledge them.

We owe it to ourselves to become as free and open to loving as possible. We can all find new sources of love both within and without. All of us can improve our ability to connect with others, as well as ourselves. Perhaps of all the adventures that await us none is as exciting and potentially fulfilling as finding new sources of love.

For those who are single or divorced it could mean an entirely new world. For those married or in a close relationship it could enhance the meaning of their lives and open doors to feelings that were never truly experienced.

What do you do if you sense a lack in your feelings, a diminished ability to love and a belief that you have become less lovable? Do you merely tolerate others and yourself rather than interact genuinely? Do you make a real attempt to change and overcome any obstacles to loving and being loved? If you decide to change, what will you do?

- The first step is striving to accept your difficulties with loving without feeling guilt or self-hate.
- The next is overcoming the belief you are unlovable.
- Finally, it is important to stop blaming others for your difficulties.

Taking full responsibility for your behavior does not eliminate the many causative factors in your past that contributed to your problems but puts the emphasis on what you do to change. At times, of course, it is necessary to pursue past events and conflicts to give you the insight to understand why you are as you are. Under certain circumstances a period of psychotherapy or counseling may be helpful.

Becoming Self-directed

To facilitate becoming more self-directed and effective in making changes in your life it is useful to write down all the negative ideas and feelings that are associated with your conflicts about love. You can refer to them as you plan exercises and programs to eliminate negativity in your life. They may include:

- Feeling empty inside.
- Fear of closeness.
- Lack of intimacy.
- A tendency to become angry when confronted by others, especially ones you allegedly love.
- Envy and jealousy of others.
- Feeling a failure in life, work and even play.
- Using alcohol or drugs when depressed or anxious.
- Feeling free only when drinking.
- Believing you haven't met the person you will fall in love with and thus it's only a matter of time and not of personal change.
- Becoming critical and judgmental when a dispute arises between you and others.

The very fact that you want to change is a constructive step. The process of change is not difficult, but does require persistence and continuing motivation. Change doesn't occur overnight, but it will happen. Believe in your ability to make it happen.

Exercises to Facilitate Change

Many of the following exercises are useful to facilitate the efforts of anyone seeking love and improved intimacy. Determine which ones apply to you and use them daily.

- Search out past experiences and attitudes that contributed to your negative self image. If you can specifically connect your feelings to experiences from the past the resulting insight frequently fosters change. Such experiences can involve traumatic episodes. You want to reduce and, hopefully, eradicate negative influences, especially from your parents, siblings and other significant people.

- At the same time begin to show a more loving and friendly side to everyone you meet. It may seem simple to smile and say good morning, but, these minor behavioral changes influence your attitude toward yourself.
- Carefully evaluate whenever you feel unloving. If someone is critical of you, a temporary unloving feeling is understandable. The feeling should quickly abate and any tendency toward being judgmental eliminated. At that point look for the positive side of the relationship and address it, if possible. If the feeling of being unloving persists, look for other reasons, especially those that are internal, such as, feeling empty or self-critical.

- With the determination to make relationships more positive try to discuss the presence of any criticalness. At times such discussions will give you insight into your behavior. An unloving person often finds reasons to be judgmental and critical, even when inappropriate. Overcoming this tendency definitely contributes to becoming a more loving person.

Sources of Insight

By consciously seeking insight into your behavior you're allowing your inner self to ferret out links to your past that will enhance your desire to change and to become the person you want to be. As you reflect on memories and experiences, you will be surprised how the mere connection you make with current behavior will often relieve pain and facilitate the motivation to change.

- Try to increase reaching out to others in group settings, such as social, educational, religious and political organizations. Such intent often brings responses from individuals who seek to befriend you. You will have created a new opportunity to overcome any tendency toward alienation or fear of social interaction.
- Love that comes from groups enhances your wish to give back in kind. Such responses enrich you. You can sense the value of such interactions and gain much satisfaction when you benefit children, the poor and the handicapped.
- Participating in political activities or working with environmental organizations to foster changes in what you believe, develops an inner sense of value and self esteem, which certainly will contribute to feeling more lovable. Since such participation tends to be shared you have engaged in activities that will bring new friends and associates into your life.

The essential element in these exercises and activities entails changing a negative belief of being unlovable and converting to a more positive belief that you are a lovable and loving person.

Fantasy and Imagination

Another important tool for overcoming barriers to love is the use of fantasy and imagination. Believe in your mental ability to change yourself and your imagination becomes a great tool of change.

You can initially take over the role of a loving person even as you seek to genuinely become loving. Play acting actually facilitates change much as an actor begins to believe he has become the role he is playing. By imagining yourself as someone who can reach out and arouse another to friendship, warmth and even love, you are setting up the inner path to make it part of your life.

Try to introduce fantasies into a relationship with someone you like and who may conceivably become someone or is someone you love. Such sharing of imagination is especially conducive to arousing ardor and playfulness in a lover or mate. Together you can take over roles of adventurers and play-act roles that you can bring into real life.

The act of taking on roles also enlivens the imagination and arouses creativity, as well as being a lot of fun. It is an effective method for older people to reconnect with their youthfulness and arouse latent and forgotten emotions. With play-acting obstacles do not exist. In time the fantasy may become real and barriers may disappear. Give it a try.

CONCLUSIONS

Overcoming barriers to finding love and friendship becomes an adventure during this new period of life. You can gain from the wisdom attained in the battles of your younger adult life. Large numbers of people who share the need of connecting to others and rediscovering love are waiting for you to find them. Through social activities, environmental and charitable groups, as well as educational venues, you will discover new friends who will expand your horizons and fill your life. Many activities await your participation that will bring new friends and lovers into your world. You have discovered new techniques and exercises to create positive mindsets. Fears of being unlovable and not being able to love will become attitudes of the past. You will have a growing belief in the power of your mind to change your life.

Chapter Four

FINDING ROMANCE

Give all to love;
Obey thy heart;
Friends, kindred, days,
Estate, good fame,
Plans, credit and the Muse,
Nothing refuse.

—*Ralph Waldo Emerson*

The hardest of all is learning to be a well of affection, and not a fountain; to show them we love them not when we feel like it, but when they do.

—*Nan Fairbrother*

Romance is a word that conjures up visions of gallant knights courting fair ladies, Camelot, elegant couples whirling around a spectacular ballroom, whispered words between a man and a woman as they steal a kiss in the soft moonlight. From such ideas movies are made and we temporarily indulge in the fantasy before us.

However, romance is real and present in every phase of life, at every age, for the very young and the very old.

Romance reveals itself in the pleasures of courtship, sexual play, nature and the extended hand of friendship. At the apex of romance's allure is the interaction of two closely connected people. The pleasure we often gain from romantic movies, even without any scenes of outright or implied sex, comes from the romantic interaction and the "chemistry" of two lovers. When the chemistry is missing, most viewers are left cold, no matter how clever and tantalizing the script.

A great romance deserves chemistry and every couple can attain it. Chemistry may be present at the very first moment of meeting and may continue for a day, a week or a lifetime. In general, it is more apt to be short-lived as the couple's period of infatuation diminishes and finally ends. However, chemistry can be reactivated or established for the first time at any age by achieving a romantic relationship and enhancing sexual desire and activity.

> *What can couples do to stir romance? Friendship, love, intimacy and sex are the cornerstones for great and lasting romances. Certainly sex can be an enjoyable act even when practiced by strangers but achieving great sex that touches a deep and abiding note within two people comes from the depth of the connectedness shared. Great sex is inextricably tied to intimacy.*

Intimacy depends on many things but to enhance romance, as well as great sex, it requires increasingly open and free communication about the thoughts and feelings that a couple has for each other. Being able to share negative, as well as positive feelings is essential to establishing true intimacy. Talking of inner conflicts, doubts, aspirations and dreams in addition to the more usual and mundane aspects of general life opens the avenue to romantic interludes. You see each other as soul mates and deep friends and lovers and sexual partners. Such communication involves exploring mutual sexual interests, feelings and behavior. Understanding the differences in female and male sexuality, anatomy and personality will give greater respect for each other's physical and mental boundaries and beliefs. All a part of intimacy.

Romance facilitates creativity. Once romance enters a relationship, two people can creatively explore expanding their personal and sexual world. I have seen couples start on a quest of discovery initiated by their romanticizing their world. They experience art, music, nature, books, movies, theater and dining differently. Whatever either enjoyed is now shared. Together they find a world of pleasure that stimulates their desire for each other.

What touched them deeply becomes part of their fulfillment. Kissing, hidden caresses, secret hiding places, singing and laughing together, looking at sunsets and just holding hands are included in their limitless palate.

> *With romance everything takes on an aura of love and contentment. Romance is ageless and is for all ages. Often older persons might actually have certain advantages over the younger adults. Through experience and much reflection they may be more aware of the wonders of romance and certainly know the kinds of barriers that might appear. They have probably pondered the times when romance had faded and what was needed to start anew. Romance is so important it behooves all of us to keep it alive and well. It needs nourishment and it needs persistence. But it can be yours.*

What are the difficulties you face in realizing such romance in your life? There are many. There's no point in pretending that achieving romance just happens spontaneously, although infatuation and "love at first sight" can stir it into existence. **Romance is a state of mind** that occurs by effort and persistence and depends on sharing your life with someone you love. You witness it in many different situations.

- Winking at your lover across a crowded room, brushing lightly, almost invisibly against each other, a quick hug and a whispered "I love you" are parts of romance.
- Smelling a flower together, holding hands as you walk down the street, hugging as you view a spectacular sunset and feeling a mutual sense of fulfillment—all fulfill the essence of romance.
- Discovering hideaways and keeping them secret.
- Having activities that are not shared.
- Weekend holidays in nearby vacation spots and romantic interludes in secluded areas where no one is present. You can find such places in parks, hidden in forests, even in the corner of a popular restaurant.
- Walking in crowded streets can be very romantic if that is a mutual intent. Looking for special objects to enjoy and possibly buy if you both loved them.
- Sending notes to each other, writing poems, finding romantic sayings or quotations that you give to each other.
- Sharing a luscious dessert in a restaurant or in your garden.

Much of what becomes romantic is based on an attitude toward each other that can be stirred by merely thinking of it. With a partner that you love the intent is quickly perceived. The interchange is stirring and creates a warmth and perhaps sexual arousal.

With such a romantic mindset it's easy to set up special dates and secret trysts. Walking into a bookstore or a museum becomes more than searching for a book or peering at paintings. It's an activity of romance, if you make it so.

- The way you speak to each other can be romantic.
- Kidding around, laughing together or having special secret ideas that are not shared with others; that's all romantic.

- Asking for forgiveness when one is out of line or inappropriately angry or annoying can be romantic; especially when two lovers ask for forgiveness from each other and end with a hug and a kiss.

In a word romance is a state of mind, a state of love, a blossoming of fervor and a kindling of an inner fire. And there's nothing quite like it to keep a couple young at heart and mind.

As currently defined, romance requires another person to share your life. Whether two people live together or only share part of their lives, romance can occur. As we age, the proportion of women to men increases lessening the chance of meeting someone. Also many people who have lived as a single person for years are reluctant to give up living alone fearing the consequences of an ill-formed relationship. Finally, two people must have the requisite compatibility to be attracted to each other.

Older people face other issues, perhaps most evident with women. One is of self-esteem and self-image. Our world overvalues youth making it appear that aging is somehow unacceptable. Women especially find it difficult to accept bodily signs of aging.

Entire industries are now devoted to offering women methods to maintain youth. Lotions, creams, hairdressers, cosmetic surgery, vitamin and herbal combinations, fashion design, support groups, books and magazines are devoted to the older woman. Self- images are modified externally with varying degrees of success. Self-esteem, though based on a sense of personal accomplishment and feeling loved by family and friends, can also be influenced by this self-image.

On another note, some women and men, particularly those who are single, feel unattractive as they age and become convinced that love and sex will elude them. Instead of finding ways to reduce their negative attitude toward aging, they tend to hide behind various activities, such as overeating, using drugs, and mainly sharing their lives with other similarly oriented people. What can be done about these feelings when they appear to be based on the reality of growing older?

First is the need to realize that such feelings are colored by the awareness of a broad-based negative attitude in our culture toward the aging person. In other cultures older people are looked up to and loved for their wisdom. The signs of aging are seen as beautiful and indicative of one's experience that comes with the passing of time.

In our culture the opposite has taken place. Certainly, many older people are revered and often held up as examples to be emulated, but this has little to do with the underlying feeling that being old is equivalent to being unattractive. Young people often have trouble imagining that their parents and other older people desire sex and romance.

Fortunately, a new trend appears to be developing. The 78 million baby boomers are beginning to enter the age of retirement and are refusing to allow old beliefs about aging to continue. As a group they are very positive and maintain a sense of youthfulness, which may be changing the negative attitudes about growing old.

Many older people are accepting their aging as part of the natural life cycle that in no way excludes feeling worthwhile and beautiful. They are developing a new mindset. **If you believe that old is beautiful, then indeed you will feel beautiful.**

Is this difficult to accomplish? For some, the answer is yes. For most, the answer is NO, but it does require breaking attitudes that have governed your life for years. Think back when you were young. Did you revere older adults and see them as beautiful and accept that one day you too would reach that age? Or did you tend to write them off and find it difficult to imagine that one day you would stand in their shoes?

By overcoming negative beliefs you will begin to actively change your view of aging. Instead of taking the passive road to getting older you will begin to find ways to live up to your growing acceptance that being older is being beautiful and deserving of the love and romance that comes with such an attitude.

EXTENDING ROMANCE INTO A TOTAL LIFESTYLE

As older people accept a more positive attitude toward aging, many find it easier to diet and exercise. Walking for fun, as well as for exercise, becomes part of a new lifestyle. There is greater pleasure in seeking new friends and joining groups. They find that life has become more romantic and discover that romance is not only between two people but between them and the world.

They become part of the bounty of nature and view things differently. They revere the aged in our world. Old trees, old beautiful buildings, flowers that last longer, ancient civilizations. Traditions of the past that brought stability and hope are readopted. They have begun to develop a loving and romantic attitude to the world about them. The world begins to look different. Some become more protective of this "new" world and join environmental groups or plant trees and flowers. Others travel more for rediscovery and exploration. They feel the pulsations of the world. They can be deeply touched. They are developing a romantic relationship to their world.

Does such an attitude translate into a romantic relationship with another person? Yes. As they begin to reveal more aliveness and vitality, they then become very appealing to others. There are millions of single people who want and desire romance and love. They only need to find each other. Even those who are married and in permanent relationships will find a new awakening together as romance enters their life.

Romance can begin to envelop you. The scope is unlimited. The path ahead will make the coming years fulfilling and happy ones. Romance has many guises and appears in ways least expected. It is how you open to the world and consciously desire to be a romantic.

How about a romance with music? We all have favorite music from our younger years. Sitting quietly in your home or attending a concert and listening intently to a Mozart concerto or a Beatles song or to Bob Dylan add a new dimension to your life. And how about seeking out new music and exploring areas that might have been bypassed? Music enlivens your world and adds a quality to life that can be repeated over and over.

The same goes with increasing your study and appreciation of art. The world is filled with museums, art galleries and libraries. Becoming immersed in understanding art that may have appeared esoteric or unappealing at one time can be both entertaining and enlightening. It can revive old interests and perhaps awaken your own creativity. Careful scrutiny of art allows you to share a vision with the artist. Isn't that a kind of romance also?

Much of romance then is a personal attitude and in many circumstances only secondarily involves a partner. What if, despite all your efforts and changes, you don't find that elusive partner? That may happen, but what have you lost? By changing your perspective about romance you have brought much pleasure and gratification into your world. You have discovered how to romance the world and yourself.

Finding ways to make your life more enjoyable and building a romantic relationship with yourself and the world can't be negative. You would have found a way to make your life better, more creative, healthier. No doubt you will attract new friends and enjoy outings and ventures with others. And you will have found yourself happier and more alive. You would have become your own romantic partner.

Have you ever tried winking at yourself when looking in the mirror? It can't help but put a smile on your face. Going for a walk alone and stopping to admire and smell the roses that you pass is a tacit connection to something beautiful that you reach out to. I consider that connection to be romantic. You definitely feel a strong emotion when you touch a rose.

> *There is no doubt that any changes that you make that add pleasure and fulfillment to your life can be thought of as romantic. Becoming a romantic will*

contribute to setting you on the path to a happier life and also to finding a partner to share your romantic life. Romance is a state of mind, an incredibly stimulating state of mind, and it is in you.

Chapter Five

IGNITING YOUR SEX LIFE

Young love is a flame; very pretty, often very hot and fierce, but still only light and flickering. The love of the older and disciplined heart is as coals, deep, burning, unquenchable.
— Henry Ward Beecher

The psychological need for intimacy, excitement, and pleasure does not disappear in old age, and there is nothing in the biology of aging that automatically shuts down sexual function.

—Williams H. Masters, Virginia E. Johnson and Robert C. Kolodny

Having a satisfying sex life is one of the prerequisites of living fully during your retirement period. It's a time for fun, relaxation and making love. Sex can be enjoyed at any age. Although there is a gradual reduction of desire and frequency for many couples as they move into the second half of life, the ability to engage in satisfying sex continues unabated. But for many, sex is no longer part of their lives. Through neglect or lack of desire or just tiredness having sex slowly declines. This chapter is dedicated to those whose sex life has ended and those for whom it is not satisfying or sufficient. There is absolutely no reason to stop having sex in your life. Hopefully with a partner. If not, engage in sex for self-gratification. Or both.

Sex may take different forms and older people can take advantage of them. We are more experienced and understanding of what offers our partners the most satisfying sex. We are more relaxed with manual and oral sex. Intercourse may become less frequent but not less gratifying. Techniques for prolonging intercourse can give new pleasures to men and women. Sex can become more than just an orgasm. It becomes a time for meaningful intimacy and may even involve a spiritual closeness.

Although there is a gradual reduction of libido and the hormonal levels that are needed for maximal arousal there is no truth that as we age we lose the ability to make love. Although men may find that their previous hard erections have become less firm, they are still very capable of having intercourse even if not as frequently. The refractory period between erections has lengthened. No more can they have one erection after another. Instead there is a greater interval of time needed for the body to recover the physiological basis for having another erection.

For many, spontaneous erections are fewer and they need greater stimulation for arousal. These factors are part of aging but in no way precludes the ability to engage in enjoyable sex. Today there are drugs, such as Viagra that are effective for erection disorders. Many men who have used Viagra find that with a better understanding of what is needed for arousal the need of such drugs diminishes or disappears.

After menopause women find that their vaginal mucosa thins and there is less vaginal secretions thus making intercourse painful. For many this tendency increases as making love diminishes. At times, even with adequate sexual frequency, the vaginal dryness is unabated. If so, there are many vaginal creams to moisten the vagina so intercourse is as pleasant as in the past.

Sexual desire tends to remain high unless the scarcity of sex slowly reduces desire. Eventually many couples and singles stop having sex altogether, except for masturbation practiced by some. This is unfortunate as the loss of sexual gratification tends to reduce self-esteem and increases the feelings of growing older. How much more desirable is maintaining the belief that retirement in its own way is a time to reestablish a feeling of youthfulness and sex should be a part of it.

I'd like to introduce you to a delightful couple who came to see me for sex therapy. What they learned during therapy is a veritable book on how to enhance your sex life during this vital period of your life. Nothing marred their satisfying life except for......well, let me tell you their story.

Despite a happy life, Rachel and Bob desired more exciting and fulfilling sex. Like most people they had fantasies and dreams of greater sexual satisfaction, but did little about it until one New Year's Eve they decided to seek sex therapy and were referred to me. It gave me an opportunity to work with a couple who enjoyed sex, loved each other, were very upbeat and wanted to romanticize their lives. They were highly motivated to try anything to bring sex back into their world.

They had no sexual hang-ups and no inhibitions, only a lack of desire that they were determined to change. And they did. You will discover with them the many ways that any couple can enhance sex, love and romance. As you follow their actual therapy sessions you will discover ways to pursue your own sexual interests.

"We came for a little sex therapy," Rachel smiled warmly after our mutual introductions. "My husband and I haven't been into sex much and we think we're missing out."

"In what way do you believe that?" I asked.

"Although we're no spring chickens, we just think we should have more sex," she laughed.

"Completely reasonable desire," I said. "Please tell me about yourselves, including your sex lives."

Rachel was a charming and attractive woman in her mid sixties. She appeared at ease sitting close to her husband and had taken his hand immediately on being seated. Bob, tall, looking younger than his 71 years, handsome and calm, seemed ready and even eager to participate in our meeting.

"Well, there isn't much to tell," Rachel said. "We've been happily married for 37 years, have no children and enjoy our jobs. I'm an accountant and Bob is an executive in a small electronics company and is on the verge of retiring. I don't have any skeletons in my closet. My parents who lived to old age had a happy life, and I have a younger sister who lives on the East Coast whom I see a couple times a year.

"Bob and I feel the same way about sex and have never had any trouble. I never had much interest in sex, even as a teenager. We still have sex about once a month and it's quite enjoyable. We just want to learn to have more sex and wonder why we don't have the same interest in sex as other people." She stopped and tapped her husband on the thigh. "Your turn."

Bob smiled and gave his wife a quick peck on the cheek. She smiled at him.

"Rachel said it all about our sex life. I was into sex a lot when I was younger and Rachel and I did have a lot more sex in the earlier years of our marriage.. However, for the last fifteen or twenty years my interest in sex has definitely dwindled. I think Rachel and I began to lose interest in sex about the same time so it's never been a problem. We just assumed it was due to our getting older.

"But we now definitely think we're missing out. And we keep reading that having a good sex life is important for health and that people are happier and it helps keep you young. That part sounds good to both of us," Bob laughed. "Actually we kind of feel that we're missing something that we still enjoy when we do have it. It's not like we don't like or want sex. We really like it.

"My family background is quite normal. My father was a gung-ho kind of guy and played basketball with old buddies. He could beat me in tennis, which he did regularly. It gave the old man a kick and I didn't care. Up until he died about seven years ago, he was still willing to take me on in tennis.

"Mom was a homebody, always had people over and spent her days cooking and taking care of my sister and me. Although she had heart disease in the last four or five years of her life she was a hearty soul when she died about three years ago. I'm close to my sister and love her two kids and their four children. Her husband and I never became friends but we tolerate each other. No problems there.

"As a gag, Rachel and I had been given a porno video for Christmas by a good friend. He had asked me what Rachel and I do for sex now that I'm thinking of retiring. When I told him very little, he just laughed. Before we knew it, we were watching a sleazy porno video. We had never watched one together and the last one I had seen was in college.

"This was actually a pretty good flick and it made us think of all the things we don't do, when we occasionally have sex. But it didn't really turn us on either. We never feel a sexual spark that makes us want to have sex on the spot. That's what the video showed. The girl wanted sex all the time and she always found men ready to trot. So Rachel and I began to talk and thought we're missing out. I agree with Rachel that we came here for some instructions on how to have a better sex life."

Sex therapy is generally brief, usually about six sessions, unless individual problems, such as excessive anger, fear, guilt or feeling unloved interfered. If so, the couple usually agreed to some couple therapy, which was generally sufficient to resolve those difficulties and allow the sex therapy to proceed. In addition, the benefits of having a good sex life following the therapy often lessened the effect of other symptoms.

"So although you weren't turned on by the video, it stirred you to wanting more sex," I said smiling. "You're not alone in finding a stimulus that motivates you to take action. How about if we start by one of you telling me about your sex life and anything else that may contribute to your current low sex drive. Since your sex interests are similar, your marriage hasn't suffered as it might have if there had been a marked discrepancy in your sexual needs."

"Should I start, Rachel?" Bob asked, while squeezing his wife's hand.

Rachel nodded and murmured, "Okay."

"I think I fell in love with Rachel at first sight. She was everything I ever dreamed about in a woman. Beautiful, smart, sexy looking, warm, easy to talk to, and we seemed compatible in everything. When I tried to kiss her on the third date, she turned her head and I kissed her cheek. I remember her saying, 'That was nice' and giving me a good hug. She said goodnight and when she went into her apartment I felt like I was walking on clouds. I knew then she was the girl for me.

"We didn't really make it for a couple of months but it didn't matter. When we finally went to bed it was great. I remember we were listening to Chopin's etudes or waltzes and after the sex we just held each other and got into the music. She was perfect and still is even though over the years our sex has just about stopped. That's the whole story. Now we just think we'd like to add more sex to our life, but our love and future would be great without it."

"How about your view of your sex life?" I asked Rachel.

"What Bob says is what I also felt when we met. Bob and I just have a way with connecting. We don't even have to talk to share ourselves. We love to listen to music together and do almost every night when we go to bed. Whenever we decide to have sex, we put on our favorite romantic music.

"I also loved Bob from the beginning. I was never into sex. When I fell in love with him, it didn't make me want to jump into bed, although I love to feel his body against me. Bob didn't mention that we cuddle and kiss a lot and love to touch each other. We also give each other massages once or twice a week. I like sex when we have it. Bob is actually a great lover. He always makes certain I come. And I always feel good. But I just don't have much interest in sex most of the time even when we're cuddling. My girlfriends say that when they cuddle and their husbands or boyfriends begin to get hard, it usually ends up in sex. That never happens with Bob and me. We just love cuddling."

"Perhaps one of you can start and describe what actually goes on in one of your sexual encounters," I said, as I reflected on their obvious happiness and their desire for sex therapy to enhance an already fulfilled life.

Bob smiled at Rachel, who picked up the cue and began. "Since we don't want sex often, we almost always plan it. One of us brings it up, usually at dinner. If the other agrees we then plan the evening. I place candles in the bedroom, put on one of Bob's favorite perfumes and bring in flowers from our garden.

"We often take a shower together. Once in bed, we caress each other and really get into kissing. Then we stimulate each other's genitals with our hands and when I'm ready, we have intercourse. Usually I've already had an orgasm. Bob is very gentle and I love feeling him inside me. Sometimes, I even have another orgasm during intercourse." She stopped and smiled at Bob.

I was definitely puzzled. From her description they seemed to have an ideal sex relationship. Bob was obviously a caring lover and even without further details it would appear he had no problems with impotence or premature ejaculation. Rachel was orgasmic, both by manual stimulation and intercourse. With such mutual pleasure I only wondered why they hadn't increased their frequency earlier.

"Bob, do you want to add anything or change anything that Rachel said?" I asked.

"I don't think so. Except, perhaps that our love making is always very romantic and I love being inside her, especially the way we do it."

"What way is that?"

"Rachel likes to be on top and I like that best too. I can then play with her breasts and we can kiss and she can move around any way she wants to try to have another orgasm."

"Your love making sounds very satisfying for both of you," I said. "You have included the romantic elements that really make it special. I am curious, however. With so much obvious pleasure you receive from love making why don't you do it more frequently? It seems that the very fact of your mutual pleasure would induce you to repeat it."

"We've thought about that ourselves," Rachel said. "We often go back to favorite restaurants and repeat favorite hikes, but not sex. Whatever we do, we want to do out of desire and not mechanically or artificially. So we only have sex when one of us really feels the need. We hope you can help us in that department."

If what they said was accurate, then my job was to help them become sexually aroused more frequently. They seemed very compatible, obviously loved each other and communicated easily and openly. Nevertheless, I still looked for less obvious reasons why their sexual desire was so limited. The usual reasons, such as anger, childhood trauma and abuse, incompatibility in their temperaments, personality differences and inhibitions based on previous conflicts with parents, didn't seem pertinent here.

"All right. Let's talk about sex therapy for you. The usual problems of erection difficulties or Rachel's lubricating adequately that affects some older people don't apply here. Although you didn't specifically address these areas, I'm assuming there is no sexual dysfunction. Plus you both enjoy and desire sex. Am I right?"

"Oh, yes," both said brightly.

"It might be helpful to your therapy if you each went over anything from your past that might be contributing to your low sex drive."

"Doctor," Bob responded, after glancing at Rachel, who nodded at him, "Rachel and I don't think it would be helpful for us to spend time telling you anymore about our past. We only want to learn about ways to enjoy sex more frequently."

I looked closely at Bob and Rachel, sitting at ease and waiting. Since sex therapy is a behavioral technique, knowledge of the past is not essential for it to be effective.

"That seems reasonable to me," I agreed. "If I feel that such information is important to our work, I'll let you know. At the moment I don't anticipate needing it. Is that satisfactory to you?"

"Sounds fine with us," Rachel answered. "So what is the first thing we do in sex therapy?"

Sensual Exercises: Mutual Pleasuring

"We'll start with a week of sensual exercises. Each day that you are both in a receptive and positive mood and desire to do the exercises, undress, and set up whatever romantic elements you want in your bedroom, much as you now do for love making. Make certain your bedroom is at a pleasant temperature.

"Take equal turns pleasuring each other with your hands. You'll caress each other, over every part of your body except your genitals. For Rachel, that also includes her breasts. Give each other the same amount of time. Bob, if you caress Rachel for twenty minutes then she would do the same for you. The important part of this exercise is that you **communicate** whatever you're doing."

"You mean we talk while doing it?" Bob asked.

"Yes," I replied. "But it's a certain kind of communication. I'll explain in a moment. To simplify my description I'll assume that Bob starts out as the caresser and Rachel is the recipient. By the way, this is caressing and not massaging.

"Bob, you can use all parts of your hand, however. Palm, fingers and knuckles. Rachel, you will tell Bob if you like or dislike what he's doing, if it feels good, wonderful, or the opposite. You can ask him to press harder or softer. You can suggest that he uses fingernails or the tips of his fingers. The objective is to discover what truly pleases you and for Bob to improve his technique to give you pleasure.

"To enhance this exercise, Bob, you should also ask Rachel, unless she's already commented, if a certain maneuver or technique is pleasurable and if you can improve it. You will find that even with your skills of caressing that there will be much to discover here. Certain areas of the body are much more erogenous and give more pleasure than other areas.

"Most lovers are surprised to discover what they find out. Anyway, you can't lose because the exercise is fun and is something that you can do as foreplay for the rest of your lives. The communication part is essential to improving other areas of your lovemaking, which we'll get into later."

"This will certainly be different for us," Rachel said. "We never talk when making love. We just go with the flow."

"Won't so much talking and analyzing every movement interfere with the pleasure of the experience?" Bob asked.

"Actually not. Once you find out about your individual responses and recognize the number of erogenous zones, which often change temporarily, then you won't want to talk. But realizing that talking enhances lovemaking and, not the opposite, is important to know. It's much like knowing what goes into a gourmet dish. It doesn't interfere with your pleasure in eating it."

"If we get through all your usual exercises with flying colors could you teach us about tantric sex?" Rachel asked.

"Why, of course, if you'd like to go into that. It's quite different from the way most people experience sex, as you probably know."

"Since we decided to make our sex life a more important part of our general life, we want to learn it all," she added.

"I'd be happy to teach you other special techniques about making sex more enjoyable, if you desire. Why don't we see how things go? Remember no genital touching this week," I said.

"No fear," Bob answered. "See you next week."

After they left, I thought how unusual they were, at least for sex therapy patients. Quite refreshing! I quickly reviewed the session wondering if there was something I missed in this apparently idyllic relationship.

They entered my office wearing big smiles. "You have no idea how great it was doing what you suggested," Bob said, as he sat down. "I never knew that Rachel loved to have the soles of her feet scratched with my finger nails. When I did it to her she almost flew off the bed."

"It was like suffering in ecstasy," Rachel laughed. "I used to think it would just make me squirm or laugh, but it's actually quite exciting."

"Well, you have discovered that there's excitement in body contact that doesn't necessarily have to lead to sex."

"We always knew that the small of our backs aroused us," Bob said, "but believe me when Rachel moved her fingers back and forth extremely slowly, I could hardly lie still."

"You had mentioned that some of our favorite places might change and you were right. The first night when Bob rubbed his hand on my inner thigh it really felt good. It was my favorite. The next night I found out that scratching my feet was best. I was also surprised when he began to do all sorts of things to my head with his hand. I really loved that. I don't think we would have felt most of what we did unless we encouraged each other to do things differently. You were right; talking about it really helped."

"Did you have an opportunity to do it everyday?"

"All but one, and they were always at night," Bob answered.

"I failed to emphasize," I said, "that you should only engage in the exercise if you're both interested in doing it. Actually, I realized that you were truly eager to learn and that would not be a problem. Normally, a couple's response to this exercise tells me a lot about their closeness, willingness to share and how much resistance I'll have as we go through the sex therapy. If a couple is unable to enjoy doing this simple exercise, I usually have to devote more time to regular couple therapy and help them overcome underlying problems in the relationship."

"What do we do now?" Rachel asked.

"We'll go over the next exercise shortly. Before we do, however, do you have any questions about your relationship or what you did last week or anything else for that matter?"

"I know I asked before, but could you tell us what tantric sex is?" Rachel asked.

"You seem quite intrigued by tantric sex."

"I just like to know what it is even if you don't teach us about it."

"I'll tell you something about tantric sex when we are near the end of your sex therapy and you have accomplished what you desire. In the meantime I suggest that you buy a few books or videos in order to gain some understanding about this ancient tradition. I believe you'll find them most interesting."

"We like to learn it all," Bob said enthusiastically.

Sensual Exercises: Genital Stimulation

"Since you thoroughly enjoyed last week's exercises, this week we're going to build on it. You do the same thing with each other and continue to communicate. Only now in addition to full body caressing you will include the genitals and breasts. In general, most couples tend to caress the body first and at the end of the exercise caress the genitals. The caveat here is that there are to be no orgasms. You learn how to enjoy sexual caressing only using the hand and attain heightened levels of arousal without coming.

"Most important is to try to **improve the way that you stimulate each other's genitals** and, in Rachel's case, breasts. Bob, when you're caressing the vaginal area, and that includes the clitoris, you need to listen closely to what Rachel tells you. And, of course, the same applies to you Rachel, when you're stimulating Bob's penis. Many couples never attain the level of excitement possible with manual stimulations because they have never told their partners how to improve their technique.

"Rachel, though you have probably tried a variety of ways to stimulate Bob, even masturbating him to orgasm, there are most likely additional things you can learn from him."

"What if one of us becomes so excited that it leads to an orgasm?" Bob asked.

"Just enjoy it. The idea is to be aroused to near orgasm and then to verbally tell your partner to stop the stimulation of your genital. In a twenty minute period for sensual caressing, for example, you might stimulate the genitals just once for several minutes. Or you may decide to do it several different times, and during the intervals caress other areas of the body. Try to experiment with different amounts of genital stimulation and see how you like it."

I frequently use this same technique with men who have erectile dysfunction problems or premature ejaculations. However, the amount of penis stimulation is generally greater and more frequent.

"In regular foreplay couples frequently alternate genital stimulation with kissing, caressing, massaging or with periods of no bodily contact. Try whatever fits into the general scheme of the exercise. Just keep in mind that you're trying to achieve increasing amounts of direct genital stimulation without having an orgasm. This exercise is one I use to help people prolong sex and intercourse in tantric sex."

"What if after a few days of this we become really horny and just want an orgasm?" Bob asked.

"In that case make love, but keep it separate from the exercise. Unlike the first week there's nothing lost if you have actual intercourse during the week. However, I would keep it to a minimum so your sexual energy goes into the exercises where you have to learn how to control having orgasms when your genitals are directly stimulated."

"Sounds like a lot of fun," Rachel acknowledged.

"It is," I assured her. "Keep in mind that when Bob stimulates your vaginal area, he is not to penetrate your vagina with his finger. It's important that he learns how to arouse you by touching the lips of the vagina and how to best stimulate your clitoris."

"Sounds like we'll be in bed all day doing this exercise," Bob said heartily.

"Just make sure you don't forget to eat and drink water," I laughed.

"How about mixing in eating chocolates or truffles?" Rachel asked.

"A little indulgence is permitted, as long as you don't replace the sexual stimulation with eating chocolates."

The session ended with Bob and Rachel almost dancing out of the office holding hands.

"It was most enlightening," Bob started, "when Rachel described how she liked to have her clitoris caressed. I never knew that she preferred to have the area around the clitoris stimulated first and not to touch the clitoris until she was already excited. Then, when it's kind of swollen to press on it firmly and not rub it too hard."

"Bob learned that the first time we did it and for the rest of the week it was marvelous," Rachel said. "My problem was to avoid having an orgasm and on two occasions I had one. But there's no doubt that I can control it. By the end of the week I was able to prevent having an orgasm no matter how excited I became. Not bad for a beginner," she joked.

"It's hard to measure up to Rachel," Bob said with a laugh, "but I was certainly hard when she got her hands on me. Anyway, I always knew that the underside of my penis was almost as sensitive as the area around the head, but I had never fully grasped how much pleasure you get when you really slow down the stimulation of those areas. When Rachel rubbed the head very slowly, I felt I was going to jump out of my skin. Not having an orgasm was not easy, but I came through the week without one during our exercises. Admittedly, we had regular sex twice during the week."

"Well that sounds as if you used two months' supply in one week," I said lightly. "You've got to be careful or you may find it difficult to get back to your old sex routine."

"That old routine is gone, gone, gone," he laughed. "How about that, Rachel?"

"I don't even remember what it was," she replied with a broad grin. "So what do we do now?"

"I need to be careful what I tell you two or you might want sex all day long. Then, before you know it, you'll have to come to see me to tame your sex drives."

Bob and Rachel laughed and gave each other a big hug. "Do you think that our loving to do these exercise is the same as loving to have lots of sex?" she asked, looking at me.

"Well, the pleasure you're both enjoying is sexual, as well as sensual, which is what stirs one's sexual desire," I said, without exactly answering her question.

"In that case we may already have the reverse problem," Bob joked.

"Well, I've never had a case where someone wanted to reduce their sexual activity, when both people equally enjoyed sex. I'm going to work doubly hard so you want sex all the time. Then you'll have to come back and offer me the chance to reduce your sex drive. Now that should be a real challenge."

Again the laughter. Behind the humor they were feeling more sexual and definitely sharing a vision of having sex much more frequently.

"Is there anything further either of you would like to share about your experiences last week?"

"I found that when Bob rolled my vaginal lips in his fingers very gently, it was very exciting. I really wanted him to stimulate me inside but we heeded your words. When he ran his fingers using the back of his finger nails down my inner thigh that was wonderful. He caressed around my nipples very slowly and that felt especially good. I already knew that slight pinching was stimulating but he also did it when he was pressing them inward.

"It's amazing how many things you can think of when you're searching for ways to make sex better. When we had sex in the past we didn't want to interrupt anything, so we rarely tried to improve what we were doing. It all felt good and I guess I was afraid of hurting Bob's feelings since he was such a good lover. I never thought of doing it together and making it fun, as we're doing now."

"Rachel's right," Bob added. "I also didn't want to interrupt a good thing. Rachel was always good at stimulating my penis but I had never told her what I liked best. This week I opened up and really had her experiment by changing how fast and how slow she'd rub the entire shaft of my penis. She had done that before but not with my directing it so carefully. Just doing that made a difference in my being aroused. What I already told you was the thing that was most exciting." Bob paused, before adding, "I was wondering how this approach will help us doing oral sex?"

"That's on our agenda," I said. "Do you both enjoy oral sex?"

"Oh, yes," they spoke in unison.

Sexual Exercises: Intercourse

"Let's see how we go. Today our focus is on intercourse. For clarification I need to ask a few questions. Bob, do you ever have any trouble maintaining an erection or having premature ejaculation?"

"Sometimes I ejaculate too quickly."

"What is too quickly in terms of actual time?"

"Well, I imagine about four or five minutes."

"Does that seem accurate to you, Rachel?"

"Yes."

"What makes you think that four or five minutes is too rapid?"

"Because it doesn't give Rachel time to have another orgasm."

"Good reason, though having intercourse for four or five minutes is not considered having a premature ejaculation. Rachel, how much time does it take you to have an orgasm through intercourse?"

"It varies, but usually about six or seven minutes?"

"Does that seem about right to you, Bob?"

"I think so."

"All right. Women show considerable variability in the amount of time needed to achieve orgasm through vaginal intercourse. Even women who do not have an orgasm that way enjoy the closeness and special intimacy that occur with intercourse.

"**Bob, you already understand that the measure of a great lover is to make certain that the woman is always satisfied first, as you do with Rachel**. If you make certain that Rachel has an orgasm by manual or oral sex before you start intercourse, your sex relationship will always be very satisfying to both of you. Certainly, at times, when Rachel feels capable of multiple orgasms during intercourse, you can forgo that requirement.

"Rachel, let's start our work for this week by **determining how Bob can make intercourse more stimulating for you**. What can Bob do to facilitate your having an orgasm during intercourse?"

"I don't know. Sometimes it happens and sometimes it doesn't."

"Is it related to how he penetrates you?"

"I'm not sure. I usually get into a position on top of him that seems best for me. He's very good at letting me position myself anyway I want."

"Have you tried other positions?"

"Yes, in the past, but I've done it this way for years."

"Are you willing to experiment with other positions during the week?"

"Absolutely."

"Do you believe that extending the time of intercourse would increase the likelihood of your having an orgasm?"

"I think so."

"All right. We'll incorporate all your ideas into the exercise. This week you have a choice to continue the exercise of last week or to extend it to having intercourse," I said. "You can even decide what you prefer while doing it. Since you may not want intercourse every night, you have complete flexibility.

"You first go through the last week's exercise as foreplay. However, this week again, you will not have an orgasm before you have intercourse. Bob, you will stimulate Rachel in the ways she likes including using your fingers inside her vagina. Rachel, do you feel stimulated in the area of the G spot?"

"I don't know. Sometimes it feels good where I believe it's supposed to be, but I've never had an orgasm there unless it's with his penis and then I can't tell."

"That's the usual experience. A woman having an orgasm during intercourse usually can't localize the site of the orgasm. The stimulation may involve the clitoris, vaginal lips, G spot and vaginal wall.

"The G spot is supposed to be about one and a half inches into the vagina on the upper or anterior surface. If your finger penetrates to about the second knuckle you're in the vicinity of it. There's still a question whether it exists for all women, and it usually isn't a distinct anatomical site unless the woman is sufficiently aroused. Then it feels like a slightly roughened area on the vaginal wall about the size of a nickel.

"Rachel, you'll know if Bob stimulates it. It's not easy to find even when a woman tries to do it herself. Bob, I suggest you probe around in that area each night to see if Rachel is reactive there. Always do it after she's been aroused by clitoral stimulation first."

"Won't my probing around interfere with Rachel's pleasure? It sounds clinical."

"Plan on doing it as part of your foreplay. Our work doesn't depend on Rachel's having a G spot, since it's a variable in women and can't be counted on. Don't spend much time searching for it. If it's not apparent in the first few times you try to find it, let it go for now. You can always search later.

"Instead, when Rachel says she's ready for you to enter her, meaning she's highly stimulated by the foreplay and is very well lubricated, she'll guide your penis into her. **The purpose of this part of the exercise is for both of you to prolong intercourse and extend your control over your own orgasms.**

"Bob, we'll start with you. Keep in mind that you do not have premature ejaculations. **This is strictly to give you greater control and eventually help Rachel have orgasms. It will also help you to extend intercourse for as long as you wish.** Initially, in this exercise, use the missionary position, that is, with Rachel on the bottom.

"Bob, continue intercourse until you feel you're getting close to coming. Then stop for a brief period. If possible, remain with your penis inside Rachel. If it gets too soft, then, exit the vagina and start the stimulation again.

"Do this a total of three times. As you try to withhold having an orgasm you will learn that you can get very close to orgasm and not have one. On the other hand, if you feel you need to ejaculate on the third time continue the intercourse until you have an orgasm. "In general, by not coming the first two times or three or even more times, you will be able to prolong intercourse before having an orgasm. Some men and women do this four, five, six or more times. As you can readily see, this is another exercise that is used in tantric sex to prolong intercourse without having an orgasm. The same technique is used with women."

"I can see how Bob's practicing to control having an orgasm will be great for me," Rachel said, smiling broadly.

"You're right," I concurred. "During all these periods of intercourse, you may have one or more orgasms."

"I'll enjoy that part too," Bob added, squeezing his wife's hand.

I smiled at their continuing enthusiasm. "On alternate nights, Rachel will decide when to stop intercourse, unless Bob is getting close and needs to stop to avoid having an orgasm and losing his erection.

"Rachel, the purpose of your controlling your orgasms is to facilitate your ability to have orgasms during intercourse, especially if it was difficult having one before. Since women can have multiple orgasms this kind of control is generally not practiced. However, by becoming more sensitive to your vaginal sensations your orgasm potential increases.

"After the third attempt to control your orgasm you can then have one, if desired. Rachel, as you practice this exercise in the coming weeks you will increase your likelihood of having orgasms during intercourse.

"By the middle of the coming week I want you both to try different positions. Here is where the experimentation can be creative. There are five primary penis to vagina positions. All of the positions used by heterosexual couples are variations of the man on top, the woman on top, spooning with the man behind the woman lying in bed, entering the vagina from the rear and the woman sitting on the man who is in the sitting position. This is one area that having a book on sex with clear pictures can show more precisely the variations in these five primary positions. However, it's not essential, since by communicating to each other you can easily experiment as you try different positions.

"For example, in the missionary position the variations are endless, depending on how a woman raises and spreads her legs. Rachel, when you try these positions you can modify them in sequence as you enjoy intercourse. You can lie flat, raise your knees, or put your knees around Bob's waist or upon his shoulders. You can have a pillow under you; your head can be elevated or flat on the bed; your legs can be spread wide or close together. All these positions can cause a marked difference in the pleasures you both have.

"Bob can move further up or down your body as he thrusts his penis into you. The further up the more likely his pelvic bone will stimulate your clitoris during his thrusting. Many women enjoy this and it often results in her having multiple orgasms.

"Experiment with as many or as few positions as you desire. The purpose is to find those ways where Rachel may more easily have an orgasm. It partly depends on stimulating the clitoral area during intercourse. As I mentioned and want to emphasize, this is accomplished by pressing the pelvic area forward when the man is on top.

"Second, is to try to stimulate the G spot during intercourse. This is generally best accomplished through entering the women from the rear, either when she is lying on the bed or when she's on her knees. The penis is pushed toward the upper vaginal wall and during the thrusting movement should stimulate the G spot area.

"At times, some women find greater stimulation when they put a pillow under them while lying on their backs. This allows the penis to glide over the upper part of the vagina. You need to experiment since the shape and position of the vagina differs with women.

"This gives you an idea of ways to experiment. It may end up that you go back to the position you already enjoy, but experimenting is useful and fun.

"Any questions?" I asked.

"That's a big order," Bob said.

"Yes, it is. I usually spread it over several or more weeks, but since you're having sex every night, follow your inclinations. Remember, if you prefer to use your favorite position and work on prolonging sex that's fine. We're in no hurry and by all means I don't want you to become frustrated by overdoing the exercises. I know I'm repeating certain things, but understanding what you expect to accomplish with these exercises is very important.

"Obviously you can't try them all this week, but it gives you an idea of what lies ahead of you after our work together has ended. During this experimental period if you become highly excited and want to go to orgasm, do so, and enjoy it. Think that's enough for today?"

"No, that's hardly a tidbit. How about learning about oral sex?" Bob said, laughing.

"Why not," I joked. "You can use it as an appetizer."

"Listen, I'm game," Rachel laughed. "We'll have sex instead of food. And oral sex will serve the old palate perfectly."

We all laughed as the session came to an end.

In the fourth session Bob said, "We followed your suggestions exactly and I found that I was able to maintain my erection much longer by the end of the week."

"Did you ejaculate when you were stimulating your penis through intercourse, when you preferred not to?"

"Not once," Bob responded. "I think it was because I never let the stimulation go too far before I either stopped or withdrew from Rachel. Nevertheless, I could handle much more stimulation, as I mentioned."

"Does that imply that you can now prolong intercourse?" I asked.

"Yes."

"Rachel, how about you?"

"I don't think I have changed. I could go a long time before, if Bob held off coming. But I found it exciting that Bob seemed to go on much longer."

"Any success in finding the G spot?" I asked.

"I don't think so," Rachel responded. "Although there were a few times when I thought it felt different when I was on top and leaning backward."

"That would tend to cause the penis to hit the front of the vagina and thus might have stimulated the G spot area."

"I gather Bob was not able to find it with his finger."

"You're right."

"Keep trying whenever you have the urge," I suggested.

"We will," Rachel replied.

"How did you enjoy trying other positions?"

"That didn't go too well," Bob replied. "Actually we spent most of the time just trying different ways of doing the missionary position and Rachel really didn't like any of them as much as the one she normally uses."

"Somehow, no matter what we did, even when Bob pushed far forward as you suggested trying to stimulate my clitoris during intercourse; I never really got turned on. I don't think trying other positions is going to work for me."

"As far as I'm concerned," Bob said, "if Rachel doesn't want to try other positions, it's okay with me."

"Many people have favorite positions, which they use all the time," I said. "The only advantage of trying other positions was to see if there were one or two alternate ways of enjoying sex together. As your sex desire increases and you want sex several times a week then occasionally you might want to try a new position. You can never be certain what might work until you try it."

"I can see the advantage of that," Rachel replied. "It would be wonderful if we both wanted to have sex several times a week. I know that I look forward to our sessions and practicing the things you tell us. I wonder if we'll still have the same desire when we stop working with you or whether we'll resume having sex once or twice a month."

The Ways of Romance: Increasing Sexual Desire

"I'm going to assume that the increased fun you've had in doing the exercises will translate into wanting more sex," I said. "But to make sure why don't we spend this session discussing how to make your sexual desire increase independent of what you do in bed."

"What do you mean?" Bob asked.

"Sexual desire stems from many things," I began. "For example, there are visual cues that stimulate men and women. Rachel, do you do anything to stimulate Bob sexually outside of touching him?"

"Of course," she said grinning. "I wear low cut dresses and show my cleavage which he likes, use his favorite perfume and I sometimes playfully do a strip tease, which really turns him on. I even walk around the house nude or just wear a towel, which I pretend is about to fall off. He knows all my tricks but he still loves them."

"You got the picture perfectly," I said.

"And what do you do to turn on Rachel outside of touching her?" I asked Bob.

"I think I'll have to learn to do a male striptease," Bob laughed. "I know that going to one of her favorite restaurants or buying her a special gift, or a single flower, or even making a pot of tea that we drink in the garden is special for Rachel. She loves when I suggest we have a drink before dinner in the living room with candlelight or a fire in the fireplace."

"Both of you are unusually romantic, which you should continue for life. It will certainly help you maintain your increased sex life. Also the things you enjoy can often be a prelude to making love. Here are a few other ideas that will help maintain the romantic feeling between you, which also may give clues that one of you is desirous of sex. I imagine you already do many of them.

In general, they all involve how you touch each other exclusive of being in bed. Hugging, kissing or making sexy physical overtures to each other at unusual times help romanticize the relationship. A few seconds of rubbing your bodies together, caressing Rachel's breast or each other's buttocks help maintain a state of expectancy for sex. Most of the time nothing will happen, but the pleasure in the contacts provides the excitement of potential sex, even when not acted on.

"Flowers, chocolates, small gifts and surprise weekends away increase romantic feelings. Occasional planning of a party for two and making love in a different place than in your home are quite romantic."

"I like all those ideas. We do some of them, but not consistently," Rachel said.

"During many nights in bed before you go to sleep," I continued, "there can be a brief sexual encounter, without it going to full sex, unless, of course, you both want it spontaneously. A real sexy kiss in bed before going to sleep often ends in a quickie, if you're both aroused.

"Reading books on sex separately or together, seeing porno films or very sexy mainstream films keep sexuality alive. Planning special sex acts, as eating food off each other, doing a striptease or exaggerated sexual dancing together can be very stimulating. In other words you're bringing sex into the relationship whenever you have an opportunity. Your natural enjoyment of sex is increasingly stimulated. People who enjoy sex often act on these stimuli and make their relationship more romantic."

"Sounds like our life will be one continuous orgy," Rachel laughed. "It should be fun and I can easily see how they will keep our sexual appetites stirred up."

"They all sound great to me," Bob added. "I wonder, though, if you think that our usual lack of sexual interest will also stop us from doing many of the things you suggest."

"Initially you have to work at it. You need to build up the anticipation and expectation of having more romance in your lives. This is where your imagination comes into play. You should both imagine what you desire from each other."

"Will that really help?" Bob asked.

"Definitely. It's often said that we are what we imagine. Having images of arousing each other, undressing each other and making love to each other facilitate wanting to have it in reality. It's actually using a fantasy to cultivate sexual desire."

"I've used images to improve my tennis game," Bob said, "It really helped."

"Why don't you practice some of these things during the week? You can continue to explore ways to enhance your sexual pleasures. Next week, perhaps, we can discuss oral sex."

They walked out of the office holding hands.

"The fun times are here to stay," Rachel said gleefully, when they returned for their fifth session. "We practiced every night, except one, and learned some important things."

"Could you tell me what they are?" I asked.

"The most important is we decided to stay with me on top and only try other positions for occasional variety. I liked most of the positions, but none really aroused me in the way I'm used to. However, I did discover that I can vary what I do on top much more than I did previously. I found that changes in my position not only affect how I am stimulated but it certainly affects Bob."

"Yes, it was quite surprising," Bob said. "Even subtle changes made a difference. Rachel tried sitting on me with her back facing me. Now that was interesting. For a few moments it wasn't comfortable until I gripped her backside to control her movements. Then it became quite stimulating, though awkward. I don't think Rachel really liked it anyway so it's probably out."

"I didn't," Rachel said. "For a short time I thought my G spot was being stimulated, but it didn't last. So it was uncertain. Anyway, I love looking at Bob and being able to lean forward and kiss him and have him fondle my breasts. I can even go all the way down and hug him. I just love doing that when I'm on top. I can also put my legs out straight and just lie on him with him in me. For me, being on top is tops."

"Sounds like your experimentation has already paid off," I said. "You can continue to experiment whenever you want. If you begin to have more sex, you may want to try new things just for fun. Some couples love to use sex toys or try positions and ideas from books on sex."

Sexual Enrichment: Oral Sex

"You mentioned that we might check out oral sex today," Bob said, winking at Rachel.

"All right," I agreed. "Tell me about your experiences with oral sex."

"I think that I speak for both of us when I say we really like it. We love going down on each other."

"It would help me to know exactly what you do to determine if there's anything that I could add to your technique."

"When I go down on Bob, which I do before we have intercourse, Bob gets very excited, as I do myself. I love to suck on the head of his penis. I run my tongue up and down his shaft and try to take as much as I can into my mouth. Sometimes, I like him to slowly move his penis in and out of my mouth, as long as he doesn't try to shove it down my throat."

"What takes place when he goes down on you?"

"I just love it. No matter what he does down there I love it. Bob is very caring and makes certain I always have an orgasm that way and I always do."

"Bob, why don't you tell me what you do to make it so enjoyable for Rachel?"

"I lick her clitoris and try to do it in different ways. I stick my tongue in her vagina, kind of nibble at her labia. I sometimes even push my nose into her vagina." He paused, then slightly flustered continued, "I can't believe I'm saying all these things to you."

"Both of you are exceptionally open and able to verbalize what you do with each other," I said warmly. "I'm certain that is why your sexual experiences were always good. The big mystery to me was why you didn't automatically want sex all the time."

"Well that's changing," Bob said. "We enjoyed all the exercises so much that we've already discussed wanting to continue having sex everyday after we stop coming to see you."

"Well," I said, smiling. "It sounds like your diminished sexual desire is a thing of the past."

"You bet it is," Bob exclaimed.

"Bob, can you describe what happens when Rachel is going down on you."

"It's great. No complaints."

"I'm curious, why you wanted me to go over oral sex since you both enjoy it and are good at what you do for each other."

"Aren't there more refined techniques?" Rachel asked.

"You may already be doing them. I'll briefly go over some of the things you can do to enhance oral sex. Remember, whenever you're trying to improve any sex technique, you must talk about what's happening and let your partner know how it feels. Otherwise, there's no way of modifying what you're doing.

"Bob, you can stimulate the area around the clitoris, the hood of the clitoris, the clitoris directly, the area between the clitoris and the vagina and all parts of the vagina. Rachel's pleasure is partly dependent on whether you're moving your tongue quickly or slowly, if you're flicking it over the clitoris, rotating it or nibbling at the clitoris. The amount of pressure you apply to the clitoris can modify the pleasure, as can the timing when you directly touch the clitoris versus when you use your tongue around it. You will find that Rachel enjoys some of what you do more than other things.

"The same goes for how Rachel stimulates your penis with her mouth. I can add a few ideas that may enhance the experience for both of you. Rachel, do you have any problem on how deep you take Bob's penis into your mouth?"

"Sometimes I gag when he goes too deep."

"That's fairly common with many women," I said. "You can control the depth of his penetration without it reducing the pleasure by forming a ring with your hand or just using your thumb and index finger. Your hand acts like your mouth and stimulates the penis, as well as controlling the depth of thrust. You place the ring formed by your hand somewhere between the head and base of the penis, wherever it is comfortable. It certainly makes it easier to give oral sex and doesn't tire you out as easily.

"Another thing to do is keep your tongue in motion when giving oral sex. Many men like the area in the back of the head of the penis stimulated. The amount of pressure, the strength of the sucking, and the rapidity of the movement of the penis in and out of the mouth will influence Bob's pleasure. The key is communicating your feelings and desires to each other. Any questions?"

Rachel and Bob merely nodded no.

"I suggest we stop here today. Unless you feel inclined to go on, we can make our last session next week. I can try and clarify any issues that remain and also go over some of the principles and techniques of tantric sex. There are no prescribed exercises so practice as much or as little as you desire. It will give you an indication of how much your sex drives have intensified during these weeks.

"We're definitely better," Rachel exclaimed as they came in for their final session. "We're kicking ourselves that we didn't see you years ago. Sex is much more fun now that we do it all the time. It's like a nightcap or dessert or sometimes an appetizer. We're having sex at different times of the day and often more than once a day. I guess we're making up for the past. We're always horny, as if we're teenagers."

Sexual Enhancement: Tantric Sex

"I see Bob nodding in agreement," I said. "Would you like to examine tantric sex?"

"We've read about it," Bob said, "And wonder if it's for us. We're not much into the spiritual stuff and only want to know how it improves sex."

"First, you must realize that it's been practiced for thousands of years and is considered a very spiritual and mystical bond between a man and a woman," I began. "It's sometimes referred to as a cosmic union between them. The emphasis is to create a bond that is sacred and rarefied.

"In traditional tantric sex a couple creates a sacred place where it is practiced. Lovemaking takes on a special glow. It's about energy flow between the participants with the ultimate joining of the yoni, the tantric word for vagina and the lingam, the tantric word for penis.

"There's a complex ritual that accompanies the lovemaking. The emphasis is on the flow and sharing of sexual energy. Whereas tantric sex emphasizes spirituality and even ecstasy we are more tuned into having great orgasms. Everything is directed to prolonging the sexual interaction, where the man does not ejaculate until the very end of the ceremonial ritual, which can go on for hours. The purpose, however, is to attain a higher and higher level of mutual spirituality.

"As you can see, such tantric sex would not sit well with the more practical and realistic American lover and thus tantric sex became westernized. Here the emphasis is also on prolonging sex, but the purpose is to intensify the orgasmic climax. However, the westernized version does retain many of the rituals, so spirituality is not ignored."

"Couldn't we just follow the westernized version?" Rachel asked.

"Indeed, you could, and you might prefer it." I replied. "My version of tantric sex is similar to the westernized form with a diminished use of rituals, but without neglecting spirituality. I do encourage lovers to take a new path to lovemaking. The path focuses on prolonging intercourse for an hour or an entire day. The emphasis is on the man not having an orgasm until the very end of the love play. It is possible for a man to learn to have body orgasms, that is, where there is a release of sexual energy, though without ejaculating. Women learn to have multiple orgasms over a prolonged period of time."

"That sounds like some of the tantric sex that I read about," Rachel said.

"It is," I acknowledged. "I imagine that the books you've been reading have thoroughly described traditional tantric sex so I won't go into it."

"We'd like to learn about your version," Rachel spoke out.

"It's rather simple, but does require a new mindset and a willingness to practice a different way of conducting your sex life. Primarily, you need to sharply reduce the usual urgency that tends to accompany sexual interaction.

"Your purpose to have a wonderful orgasm is retained but the method of achieving it is different. Everything is slowed down. Foreplay and intercourse are prolonged; there are periods of not doing anything except holding hands or lying alongside each other and not moving. Caressing each other is very slow and arousing each other takes on a new color. Frequently you have intercourse without having orgasms.

"In an earlier session I had mentioned that several of your exercises were used in tantric sex."

"Actually they were quite stimulating by themselves, especially having intercourse," Bob said. "Each time I had intercourse but did not have an orgasm my stimulation intensified. I have since found that it has definitely given me greater staying power during sex."

"Good," I commented. "You already recognize that by changing ways of having sex you have increased your pleasure in sex. **One of the primary purposes of tantric sex is to achieve increasing arousal without orgasm.** It is possible with much practice to reach a state when you experience a great release of sexual energy, which some call body orgasms, without having an ejaculation. However, achieving your orgasmic release should be very fulfilling."

"Is it really better than just having a great orgasm with regular sex?" Rachel asked.

"Not necessarily better," I replied. "Rather it's more accurate to **see the orgasm in tantric sex as fulfilling different needs and allowing a couple to share a more spiritual form of intimacy."**

"From what you say, if we just slow everything up and not rush our sexual interaction we would eventually achieve what you're telling us," Bob said.

"That's essentially true," I agreed.

"What else differs in your version?"

"It's your   mindset. You are not only doing this to achieve orgasm. You are doing this to increase your spiritual and loving connection to each other. Sharing sex this way is a blending of spirit and emotion that is distinctly different. Your fantasies are different. You try to achieve some blending with a higher spirit. You nurture the quiet moments and focus on how simple experiences affect you. You learn that merely touching each other, even just touching fingers or perhaps enjoying a very prolonged kiss, a kiss that may last for ten or twenty minutes without seeking an orgasm arouses you differently.

"You might run your finger down each other's back, but instead of taking a few seconds to do it, you might take several minutes. By totally concentrating on such an act you will both have a unique experience."

"Why would that be different from our normal ways of touching each other?"
Rachel asked.

"Because of your concentration on the repetitive action. You feel an immersion with each other that rarely occurs normally. I'm aware that what I'm saying are just words but there's no way of being more specific. You need to try it. It doesn't take long to sense the uniqueness of the experience. After several months your focus and concentration can attain a height that you never deemed possible. Your pleasure will be commensurate with your efforts to achieve that state."

"Might we become tired or bored when it appears that nothing is happening?" Rachel asked.

"If the experience bores you, then by all means don't do it. There are no fixed patterns or requirements to achieve the kind of tantric sex I'm describing. Some people find that even trying tantric sex for a short time improves their sense of togetherness. It opens their minds to a different kind of intimacy.

"If you go ahead, then your own imaginations will guide you. If your purpose is to elevate your intimacy to a new and mutually satisfying level, you will find the way of doing it."

I stopped and noted the puzzled looks on their faces.

"What do you think of this alternative way of enjoying sex?" I asked.

"It sounds rather formidable," Rachel said. "I don't know if I'd have the patience to go through it when I already enjoy having orgasms, lots of them."

"There's no reason that you can't have multiple orgasms using tantric sex techniques," I responded.

"But it seems an awful lot of work to achieve something I already have," Rachel countered.

"Perfectly legitimate point of view," I acknowledged. "It's sometimes better to see tantric sex as a different way of sex, a different method of achieving increased intimacy and a way to bring spirituality into your sex life. The entire experience has to make your love life better or why do it. And it doesn't mean that you can't use tantric sex techniques occasionally for a change of pace."

"Well, as I see it, we can't lose. If we don't like it or we're bored or it's not making our sex life better, we'll stop," Bob said

"And Bob," Rachel said. "We may find that it's helpful to our seeking a more spiritual life in addition to a different kind of sex."

"Okay, I'm for trying it and it may help me understand exactly what having a more spiritual life is all about," he said.

"Since most people separate their spiritual life from sex, you can have the best of both worlds," I said encouragingly. "At any rate anything you do to increase your desire for sex is going in the right direction."

I noted that Bob reached over to take Rachel's hand and pressed it to his chest.

"Is there anything else you'd like to discuss before we stop?" I asked.

"We've loved working with you," Rachel exclaimed. "You opened our eyes to so much and it's made our lives so much more enjoyable."

"I've enjoyed sharing your new venture into making your life more sexual," I said warmly. "However, you must give yourselves the real credit for what you accomplished. You had already developed into good lovers and only needed a little encouragement and some guidance to rev up your sexual desire. I certainly want to wish you well and that you find the fulfillment you seek."

One month later I received a letter from Rachel. One part of it told the story of what they had accomplished as they searched for ways to improve their sex life.

"Last night while lying in bed, Bob and I were holding hands listening to Mozart. I suddenly felt very lustful. Instead of acting on it as I now do regularly, I placed my hand on Bob's forehead. Without my saying a word I knew that he understood my message. Together we put our entire consciousness into the music and, at the same time, I felt my hand press deeply into Bob's head.

"For several minutes I actually believed that my hand had become intertwined with the music and had entered Bob's mind. I began to cry for at a certain moment I believed that I had become part of him and we both had become part of some universal energy.

"I know this may sound kind of crazy, but, on the other hand, I believe it was what you were trying to tell us. As our minds opened and we let our imagination soar, Bob and I reached into a world that we never knew existed. Our world has truly changed in ways we never imagined. I think that in a certain way we have combined our sexuality with a new sense of spirituality, at least what we think of as spirituality."

REFLECTIONS

Many of the ideas and techniques that Rachel and Bob integrated into their sex life are useful for everyone. Establishing romance and sexuality as a fundamental part of your life will add vitality and intimacy to it. **Realizing**

that sex doesn't always mean going to bed but, instead, becomes a way of interacting with your partner, will change your life.

Rachel and Bob epitomize what an older couple can accomplish as they enhance their love, intimacy and sex relationship. Although they came to see me without any major obstacles to sexual enjoyment their paucity of desire left them unfulfilled and certainly not fully enjoying the fruits of their later years.

Many older people do not enjoy the special pleasure that comes from sex. Whether it is due to a specific sexual problem, such as impotence, premature ejaculation, diminished vaginal lubrication, pain on intercourse or poor self-image, the result is almost always less sex, until, all too frequently, a couple stops making love.

Having sex in our older years is not only feasible but highly desirable. As Rachel and Bob learned, enjoying frequent lovemaking enhanced the overall level of their love and closeness. Once they romanticized their relationship it became a way to be together. There was no going back for them and this is true of others who achieve this heightened degree of intimacy.

What does a couple do when faced by a specific sexual dysfunction in addition to a diminished sex drive? Today there are effective drugs, such as Viagra, to help men with erection problems, which also helps many men overcome premature ejaculations.

Many of these sexual dysfunctions can be overcome, or at least improved, through the exercises described for Rachel and Bob. A strong effort to enhance sex and a willingness to do the exercises frequently results in much improvement. Even those who enjoy a satisfying sex life are more than likely not getting the degree of satisfaction possible.   Frequency may be insufficient; there may be a lack of satisfactory foreplay and the end-play may be inadequate to satisfy either partner fully.   Under such conditions sex desire diminishes and satisfaction is curtailed. Eventually, interest in sex wanes and may lead to a disorder of sexual desire. The clinical case of Rachel and Bob was such a case, although not typical, since they actually enjoyed sex once a month. With a true disorder there is little, if any, interest in sex and little or no pleasure from the act.

For women who need additional lubrication, Astroglide or Kama Sutra, two water- based vaginal lubricants, are extremely effective. For most lovers the use of these sexual lubricants enhances the pleasures from manual and vaginal sex. Putting a small amount on the clitoral area and labia increases a woman's response to manual stimulation. I have found that many women are capable of achieving multiple orgasms using these lubricants during lovemaking. Likewise, a few drops on a man's penis increase the ease and pleasure during manual stimulation. The lubricants are a valuable adjunct to sex. Because they are essentially tasteless they don't preclude oral sex.

We live in a society that abounds in sex. Sex pervades movies, books, magazines, TV, humor, fashion and invades our mind with fantasies, images and impulses. Yet a large percentage of the population either avoids sex, has less than satisfying sex, infrequent sex, or no partner.

Some believe that losing your sex drive is a natural consequence of aging. Others believe that sex and its promotion is for the young population. Advertising with its emphasis on sex is replete with young female and male models. Movies tend to star younger actors and actresses. This is certainly true for women. Less so with men. Thus once we become older, even by the age of forty or fifty, and, at the latest, sixty or seventy, sex is seemingly out of our reach implying that sexual desire has diminished as a consequence of aging.

Nothing can be further from the truth. Sex does change over the years but the desire tends to continue indefinitely. Much goes underground and is hidden in the sexual fantasies of older people. But it has not disappeared.

In recent years many polls have attempted to gather the truth about the sex experiences and habits of older people. Many indicate that a large proportion of men and women, even those who are married, but especially single older persons, no longer have sex and imply that many no longer desire it. There may be some truth in those statistics, but it takes very little to reawaken the underlying sex drive that exists in all of us.

Both men and women in their seventies, eighties and nineties can be aroused sexually when meeting an attractive and stimulating person or by maintaining a romantic relationship with a life partner. The arousal of sexual desire can certainly lead the couple to having sex. This occurs even if they have not been sexual for many years.

Older people who have found fulfillment in other areas during their older years bring to a sexual relationship experience, patience, kindness, humor, knowledge, less impulsiveness, a willingness to please, greater acceptance and a willingness to ignore or rectify areas of incompatibility. They have the ability to compromise and a desire to share love.

Having an enjoyable sex relationship may become the impetus to change other aspects of a person's life. Sex enhances vitality, is fun, improves a love relationship, is good for physical health and even leads to a longer and healthier life.

CONCLUSIONS

Sex is for all ages. Older people have many advantages in the sexual arena. They have experience, better understanding of the opposite sex, patience, time for greater romance and the wish to remain young at heart and body. With a youthful spirit, all problems and conditions that might contribute to a lessening of one's sex drive and sexual interests can be reduced and even overcome.

How often you have sex or how quickly men can have erections or women can attract men are not prime considerations. Self-esteem is based less on sexual prowess and more on personal attributes and the development of an enriched life. By communicating freely with your lover about your sexual relationship, you can increase your intimacy and so enhance your sexual and romantic life. This delightful interchange will open up new adventures and be a major component in your journey to transform your life.

Chapter Six

THE AGE FACTOR

We come to love not by finding a perfect person, but by learning to see an imperfect person perfectly.

—Unknown

If you asked me what I came into this world to do.
I will tell you: I came to live out loud.

—Emile Zola

Major age differences between partners can occur during any period of life. But perhaps they are most relevant when one of the partners is in or entering retirement. When two people fall in love they generally do not evaluate the impact of their age difference. If it had been a negative factor in their meeting, it is unlikely they would have fallen in love.

This does not imply that they were unaware of the age difference. Rather it more likely indicates that it was relegated to a place of minimal influence. Only in retrospect, at a later time, do partners assess their ages among the various factors that determine the viability of their relationship. If the relationship fails and they look for the causes of the breakup, it is likely that their age difference would be seen as one factor.

We live in an age-conscious land. Youth is eulogized and envied. It is equated with sexual attractiveness, enhanced creativity and athletic prowess. Men and women go to great lengths to avoid the feeling and appearance of aging.

To maintain the sense of youthfulness, older men have long pursued young women as sex partners and for marriage. Many young women, who seek older men for financial security, more mature sex, and the love of a father figure, welcome this pursuit. Older men tend to provide an entrance into prominent social venues, offer increased travel opportunities and, if desired, political and business connections.

In recent times, older women, especially those who have successful careers and social prominence, are drawn to younger men. Many of these women postpone growing old by accentuating their sense of youthfulness. Also, their desire for more frequent and exciting sex plays a part in seeking young men.

Younger men likewise are attracted to older, sophisticated women who manage to retain their beauty and attractiveness despite their age. Such attraction may involve seeking love missed in childhood from an absent or unloving mother. Some younger men also marry older women for financial security or even to gain control of wealth.

Frequently behind these motives and reasons to marry, even when the age difference is excessive, lie genuine love and the wish for friendship. The excitement of romantic love and the idealization of the loved one can still take place. Certainly, significant age differences can exist in great love relationships. Many older people have brought much happiness and satisfaction into their lives by marrying a younger person.

In seeking new friends and new lovers during the retirement period, marked age disparities can occur. At least one of the partners will be in their 60's or older giving considerable latitude for the age of the other. It's a time when marked age differences matter much less than previously. A man of 45 who marries a woman of 25 hardly merits a yawn nowadays. Age differences, as well as ethnic, racial and color differences, are increasingly common and acceptable to the public.

However, when a man or woman of retirement age marries a much younger person many new and significant factors enter the relationship. One person may not be working, new illnesses may develop in the older person and physical ability and stamina are not the same in different age groups. The ages of respective children can create difficulties. Different interests, often age related, may play a part in the compatibility.

There are a number of factors that influence older people to seek younger companions and to ignore the more likely compatibility of a similarly aged partner. Many older men and women seek younger partners as a way to hold on to their youth. Conversely, younger people seek older partners for security, stability and devotion. When such couples fall in love they often initially ignore the incompatibility that comes with a marked age difference. Love between two people, at any age, is generally a wonderful part of life, but alone doesn't guarantee happiness or compatibility. Couples, once beyond the starry-eyed infatuation period, attempt to assess their compatibility as more mature love is evolving. Sometimes the early bloom of love has hidden underlying problem areas that later might cause stress and even marked incompatibility. At times a marked age disparity fits into that category.

Couples with a clear age difference may be very similar in terms of attitude or mental youthfulness, physical interests, humor and seeing the world with the same perspective. Or the opposite could occur that is often not initially perceived. A case in point might be represented by a couple I saw.

The first words that Bruce said after introductions were made in their first premarital counseling session were, "Doctor, I want you to know that Clarisse is not as young as she looks. I don't want you to think that I'm some old man trying to hold on to his youth by marrying a kid. Isn't that right, honey?" he smiled, turning to his fiancée.

"Of course, darling," was her rather quiet response.

Such an introduction would immediately make me think of exactly what he was trying to deny. What it meant remained to be seen. Bruce was 68 and Clarisse was 39. He had been married once, had two children and divorced over 15 years ago. She had never been married. After almost a year of dating they decided to get married despite obvious problems that had already surfaced.

"Doctor," Clarisse began, "Bruce and I have some serious difficulties. The main reason I called you to see us is that I want children and he doesn't since he has two daughters my own age and three grandchildren. I realize I'm getting older and if I don't have them now my time will be over. My mind is not fixed on this since I love Bruce and I think I'll get along with his children, but having children is important to me.

"I want to do many things that no longer interest him and he's reluctant to give me the freedom to do them. For example, I was invited to attend a musical just last week with several girlfriends and he didn't like the ideas of my going without him to such an event. He felt that there would be a lot of single men there who would be attracted to me. I was unable to assure him that would never happen so I didn't go."

"Clarisse," Bruce broke in, "you know that one of the girls you're going with is always trying to pick up men. You've told me that yourself."

"But not when she goes out with her girlfriends. After all, Roz is married and wouldn't do anything and she's going with us."

I decided to intervene. "Clarisse, what did you mean when you said, you thought you'd get along with his children?"

"Well," she replied hesitantly, looking over at Bruce who sat unmoving. "Well, you see, I only met one of them so far, Monica, the younger one who is unmarried, and she doesn't know how serious our relationship is."

"Does she know that you're engaged?"

"No."

"Has something interfered with your meeting his other daughter?" I continued.

"She lives in Sacramento and hasn't visited us. She has the three kids and is quite busy."

What unfolded as I came to know this couple better was a number of age related problems such as the one described. Clarisse was indeed an attractive and appealing woman and an insecure man might be jealous if she sought activities without him. His insecurity could impede her freedom. I learned that he was embarrassed to let his daughters know of his wanting to marry Clarisse and in fact hadn't introduced her to most of his friends for the same reason. He avoided going out where he might be seen with her. Having children was an important reason for Clarisse wanting to get married and it appeared he had no intention of having more children. Clarisse was holding on to a fantasy. Also, it appeared that their sexual relationship had diminished to once or twice a month.

Clarisse wanted to take up tennis and Bruce felt he was too old to participate and discouraged her. Her interest in hiking and visiting national parks and Europe where she had never been was also discouraged. Bruce had traveled the world and had little interest in hiking or sports in general and travel no longer held appeal for him. He was an engineer, recently retired and spent his days reading stock charts, hoping to make his fortune speculating.

As their counseling continued, Clarisse became stronger, more secure and made more demands for lifting many of the restrictions in their relationship. His attempt to introduce his fiancée to his younger daughter was a fiasco as she refused to recognize such a union. Rather than stand up for Clarisse he tried to minimize the nature of their relationship leading Clarisse to believe he would never protect her from the demands of his children.

Over a number of sessions their incompatibility became more evident and Clarisse no longer accepted the restrictions she had previously endured. Bruce came to recognize that his need to retain his youth, have a sexually attractive companion and a woman who would be dependent and subservient had been the driving force in his love for Clarisse. Once it became clear that their relationship had little in common they graciously ended it.

At the end of their counseling I encouraged Bruce to consider meeting women closer to his age. Whether he followed my suggestion I never found out.

Marriage between people with disparate ages is fairly common and many produce happy families. In terms of overall success, providing the disparity is not excessive, there's little difference from most marriages. For Bruce and Clarisse the disparity was 29 years, relatively large and was clearly playing a part. Resolution, however, was not impossible if they had reached a common understanding about having a new family and Bruce realized that Clarisse had entered a new phase of her own life and needed encouragement to grow and find herself through exploration and new experiences.

Initially they loved each other without restraint and only with the passage of time did they recognize the conflicts and obstacles before them. By seeking therapy they came to understand some of the underlying reasons for their relationship failing. If Bruce had agreed to have children they probably would have gotten married, not entered counseling, and the other areas of incompatibility would not have surfaced until later.

REFLECTIONS

Does this imply that marriages and long term relationships with marked age-mismatched couples are doomed to failure or unhappiness? Not necessarily. Since the ingredients for most successful marriages are variable no one can safely predict which relationships will eventually work out. Much also depends on why a relationship with marked age differences develops. In general, the greater the differences in age the more likely that dissatisfaction will arise.

When age differences are extreme, as with Bruce and Clarisse, a sharp disparity in interests, energy, life experiences, knowledge and sexual desire can erode such relationships. When these differences are not understood and there is a failure of adaptation where individual needs are not met, frustration and anger can appear. Over time many such relationships fail.

Most important is not ignoring obvious and potential problems. Facing the differences and seeking solutions generally allow the development of a successful relationship. The age factor, though often pivotal in relationships, does not have to undermine mutual love between two people. Rather than one's calendar age becoming the determining factor, the partner's physical and mental age is more apt to set the tone for the relationship.

One Partner in Retirement

When one of the partners reaches the age of retirement, new conflicts may surface. The couple must anticipate them. The older partner may become bored as he leaves the work force, especially if he has not developed additional interests. He may develop more frequent illnesses, become less physically active and have decreased sexual desire. The potential of the older partner dying becomes increasingly likely giving rise to fear of loss and loneliness.

When facing these differences, awareness and communication provide the antidote for any negative factors that might arise. Recognizing and accepting that the younger person may begin to lead a more independent life will help prevent conflicts developing. Fostering the important separate activities of the younger partner generally contributes to a strong foundation for the continuing relationship.

Likewise, with adequate motivation and understanding, the older partner can take advantage of the energy and interests of his younger mate and be stimulated to find new meaning in life as he continues to participate more fully with his partner. By realizing that the activities of a younger person are well within the domain of most older people, provided that the age difference is not excessive, there need be little reduction in participating in activities together. Many people discover as they grow older that age is strictly a number and has little to do with well-being, vitality and fulfillment.

> *Love can transcend most boundaries*
> *and obstacles placed before lovers of*

sharply disparate ages. Coming from
different races, ethnic groups, religions,
or the same gender will not deter two
lovers bent on consummating their
relationship. The same is true for age
differences, no matter how excessive.

To maintain and stimulate love, when major differences exist, a couple needs to understand how to minimize this disparity. By changing attitudes, feelings and behavior toward the loved one a person can avoid the breakdown of the relationship. If the age difference becomes a greater burden than a couple can tolerate, it should be faced before it leads to increasing frustration and anger. Some relationships can't overcome this difference, much as they can't overcome other kinds of mismatching and incompatibility.

Adaptability, Acceptance and Problem Resolution

How can couples avoid having major age differences destroy their relationship? Most important is openly admitting to each other the multiple factors behind their attraction for each other and reestablishing intimacy. There is no point in hiding from underlying reasons and motivations if the marriage is breaking down. Love is the binding force and may be compromised by hidden or unspoken reasons for having established their relationship.

Adapting to the physical and mental needs of one's partner is essential for any relationship to remain solvent, especially during the older years and when there's a marked age difference. Both partners must adapt to the other. This may not be as simple as it sounds since the problems may have arisen from the disparity in interests, as well as the physical and mental differences.

We saw how Clarisse finally realized Bruce's unsuitability as a partner when she perceived his inflexibility and his refusal to accept her newly discovered need for adventure. If Clarisse had been determined to preserve the relationship, she would have had to accept becoming more sedentary and giving up her adventurous spirit. Her personal needs and newfound freedom made that unacceptable.

There are many paths that a couple can take as they adjust to one another, depending on their desires and what will ultimately give them the most satisfaction. Adaptation to the changing conditions of any marriage is one of the crucial benefits of remaining open to each other. The preservation of intimacy is at the heart of two people remaining close and loving.

A couple must determine what obstacles obscure the desired closeness before they can overcome them. If a partner refuses to make the required effort to remove barriers after they have been accurately pointed out, the relationship usually deteriorates. Bruce's refusal to try to establish a meaningful relationship between Clarisse and his daughters contributed to their breakup.

A couple knows when the relationship with a partner is not accepted by parents, children or friends and directly works to overcome this problem.

Diet, Exercise, Family and Education

A couple with a major age difference can have vastly different diet and exercise interests and needs. If the older person requires a special diet because of an illness or late-life diabetes, the younger person needs to adapt. The same with exercise. There could be a vast difference in the stamina and motivation for exercise or sports in the two people. In general, these two issues do not have to create obstacles if the two people are flexible and are willing to accommodate to each other's needs.

The same goes for differences in educational and entertainment interests. Older people, who are retired with time on their hands, are frequently more open and more motivated to seek additional education and different forms of entertainment. Generally, compromises and sharing each other's interests tend to resolve any problems that may arise in these areas. With compatible couples, regardless of age, these differences add excitement and fun to their lives.

Another conflict that may arise occurs when one of the partners has a great interest in family gatherings and sharing more with children and grandchildren. This problem is by no means confined to older people. Again with more time at their disposal the older person is inclined to be more involved with their children and grandchildren. The younger person may, at times, see this as intrusive and interfering with their personal and romantic needs.

If differences arise, the problems need to be quickly resolved. This is a sensitive area, especially if only one of the partners has children. Compatibility here is generally essential for a successful relationship. Fortunately, despite the age differences, both partners usually have children and tend to find compatible interests in each other's children, if jealousy and control issues don't erupt.

Reducing the Age Factor

Diminishing the influence of the age factor in relationships depends upon the openness and intimacy of the couple. Certainly, as with any area of incompatibility, communication often leads to resolution of the differences. Though there are many advantages for couples who are close in age and experiences; age differences do not have to interfere with developing a happy and fulfilling relationship.

Partners who want their relationship to be highly satisfying will do everything possible to augment that desire. The older partner will do whatever it takes to maintain a feeling of youthfulness, mental alertness, physical capability and health. Thinking young involves both partners. The older person needs to believe in striving to overcome the actual effects of aging. The younger partner needs to accept that growing older does have its complications and can create differences that may affect the relationship.

With effort and understanding their relationship can flourish.

CONCLUSIONS

Age tells little about the compatibility between two people. Compatibility is determined by sharing, intimacy and meaningful communication. Other significant elements include vitality, alertness, adventurousness and humor. Humor stands out.

More crucial is a couple's openness to learning, changing, growing and **sharing** core elements in their relationship. Core elements include whatever each partner strongly believes in or enjoys and has incorporated in his or her life. A strong love of music, sports, art, nature and books are important to many. The desire for romance, a strong sex drive, religious beliefs and a deep interest in politics can be core elements. Sharing core elements definitely strengthens most relationships.

Age differences need not interfere with developing a loving and intimate relationship, if the core elements are in sync.

Chapter Seven

THE PARENT CHILD LINK

Your children are not your children. They are the sons and daughters of Life's longing for itself. They come through you but not from you. And though they are with you, yet they belong not to you. You may give them your love but not your thoughts. For they have their own thoughts. You may house their bodies but not their souls, For their souls dwell in the house of tomorrow, which you cannot visit, not even in your dreams.

— Kahlil Gibran

For many retirees, the relationship with their adult children and grandchildren stands in the foreground of their retirement period. Adult friendships take the place of the previous more interdependent parent-child relationships. Equality, unfettered by the age differences, gives rise to the potential of a new kind of intimacy. Discussions, sharing old and new experiences, vacations together and planning for the children to assume greater responsibility for their parents as aging continues, if needed, are part of the developing closeness.

Grandchildren enter the picture and offer new and loving connections that fill the lives of many seniors. Grandchildren also gain immeasurably from the love and closeness of grandparents who are not involved in the actual raising of the child. For many seniors, family ties provide the most meaningful relationships they have during this final period of their lives. Although friends, spouses and frequently lovers are part of their lives the connection to their children and grandchildren usually ranks highest or, at times, second to spouses. Activities that can help maintain or improve family interactions will serve all members of the family.

Improving Family Relationships

We spend our entire lifetimes in families, starting in our childhood and ending when we're the oldest member of our current families. Thus we would think that we all know how to proceed to make our family ties as close and enjoyable as possible. However, problems appear at times that sometimes threaten the fabric of family ties.

I would like to suggest that you create another journal or use the one you might have already started to keep track of planned activities with your children and grandchildren. You might have different or separate plans for each of them and keeping a list would be helpful. Also as experiences evolve you might want to use the journal as a kind of diary of your thoughts and feelings. Since there are almost countless activities possible with your family, creating a list (see below) may provide a useful guide of family interactions.

Sometimes family get-togethers remain limited to dinner, watching television, perhaps playing a few games and maybe taking a walk. But there are many other things that you might want to consider for these family meetings, which can enliven the gatherings and also deepen them. Depending on the ages of the children and also the grandchildren these ideas can be modified. Here are a few suggestions:

1. Drawing and painting pictures together.
2. Sculpting in clay, Play Doh or Paper Mache.
3. Selecting specific topics to discuss giving the grandchildren equal time.

4. Selecting specific movies, documentaries or television specials, such as undersea creatures, watching the lives of various animals, watching movies of computer created dinosaurs, history subjects and other pseudo-educational subjects. Once kids get over the feeling these shows will be boring they often love them, and they become even more special when shared with grandparents and parents.

5. Taking the family to a special restaurant they have never been to.

6. Spending several evenings as a family planning a weekend trip for the entire family and doing "homework" to become acquainted with what lies ahead. Even if this is done once a year it is the discussion that intrigues grandchildren.

7. Taking turns reading from a children's book. Depending on the ages of the grandchildren, children can also read to the attentive grandparents. The Harry Potter books have fared well in this venture for older children. Sometimes reading books with different characters allow each person to read the lines of one character. This usually means having a number of the same books handy but this activity could go on for several or more weeks until the book is finished.

8. Sharing music. Folk music, especially Pete Seeger for all ages, rock for older grandchildren, classical music that will appeal to all family members and family participation enjoying sing-a-long music.

9. Having a drumming jam session with the family. There are a number of different kinds of small drums that are inexpensive and easy to use. The Djembe is a popular, lightweight African drum that comes in many sizes. The DhoLak , a Northern Indian drum provides another sound quality and has skins on both sides. Bongo drums are another alternative drum. Drumming is fun and can also be enjoyed solo.

10. Playing games, such as Scrabble, Monopoly, checkers, even chess.

11. Discussing politics and the environmental issues that children often find fascinating. You'll find that even younger children are more aware of political situations than

you sometimes believe. They not only hear their parents talk but they read newspapers and watch television.

12. Playing games to develop your grandchildren's creativity. (See chapter on creativity.)

Many of these experiences encourage children to become more independent, curious, freethinkers and have a sense of equality with adults that bolsters their development. By feeling the respect of their grandparents, children gain a strong sense of self-respect that nurtures their integrity and becoming self-directed.

The relationship with our adult children can be rather complex due to the many elements that are present in their personality and behavior. We are all composites of genetics, childhood experiences, traumatic events, inborn sensitivity, intuition, and that elusive element we might call chance, such as, being in the right place at the right time. Some children seem to be a "chip-off-the-old-block" and others seem to have come from a different family. Whom our children marry, where they choose to live, the kinds of work they do, all contribute to how they relate to the world and especially to their family. Although we all wish for loving relationships, at times they can be strained, distant, non-loving and even non-existent.

How do older people cope with obstacles that prevent their enjoying the fruits and delights of closeness to their children and grandchildren? It requires a bond of trust and mutual caring with children. All children want love and guidance, no matter how they might seemingly rebel. Yet the histories of families that struggled to maintain a trusting and loving environment for their children are often filled with conflict. How often voices are stilled, and children, now grown, live behind a barrier that separates them from their parents. Frequently parents are uncertain what caused the breach that only became apparent when the children left home.

An older couple, who epitomizes the struggles of many seniors, had given up on ever having a loving relationship with their daughter and granddaughter. They came to see me as a last resort.

Ben and Grace seeking a way to reconnect with their estranged daughter sought help. Marilyn, their only child, had withdrawn from the family shortly after she left for college. The estrangement had increased with the birth of her only child, Beth, now five. Marilyn and her family lived in Oakland.

Although they had first glimpsed Beth shortly after her birth, there was little contact during Beth's first year. Marilyn made no effort to either visit LA or invite them to come north. During the next three years Ben and Grace visited Marilyn and her family a few times a year. The visits were cursory, short and neutral. There were no spontaneous periods of fun and laughter. Beth enjoyed their visits and was delighted by the gifts they brought with them, but no real bond was forged and the visits were quickly forgotten once Ben and Grace returned to LA. Marilyn never visited them. The separateness had become fixed and appeared inviolate.

When Beth had reached five, Ben and Grace had come to a place in their retirement when the pleasures from their various activities had reached their apogee and a previously unrealized loneliness threatened their peaceful existence. Almost on a whim they took the suggestion of an older woman whom I had previously seen in therapy and called me.

Ben and Grace learned how they had inadvertently jeopardized their relationship with their daughter by too frequent trips during her childhood that did not include her and general neglect by allowing servants and nannies too much control. Busy most evenings, they avoided those special bedtime stories and hugs that children love. Marilyn developed a fantasy world with imagined friends, which her parents welcomed as another activity that would keep Marilyn busy without her parent's involvement. Ben and Grace did not participate in activities with the parents of other children causing Marilyn to feel more isolated and less able to make friends.

The case of Ben and Grace represents many of us. We try to do the best we can as parents but frequently are unaware of the reactions of our children. Children are far more sensitive and aware than we realize. They often hold their true feelings inside. When they finally take leave of their childhood home and take charge of their lives, alienation and estrangement from their parents can result. Such separations almost always negatively influence both the parents and the children, and it behooves all parents to overcome the barriers that prevent their forming a loving and close relationship with children and grandchildren.

How many times have I seen parents look back on their past and regret certain acts, especially those that hurt their children. No explanation can satisfactorily counter their guilt and regrets. They needed to forgive themselves and search for ways to make up for the past and establish a new and more loving bond with their children.

> *Although one can't change the past or the memories of events that affected any of us, we can modify our inner reactions, such as guilt, having a sense of badness, being overly critical toward ourselves and feeling unworthy of being loved. Such changes are more readily accomplished by making amends, looking for forgiveness from those you have injured, forgiving those you believed injured you and above all forgiving yourself. Forgiveness relieves inner pain and fosters the redevelopment of love.*

If family members are able to reconcile and bring back joy and love, the past is quickly forgotten. People are rarely made of stone and inwardly hope to find a way to resolve the conflicts that have taken away love and devotion. Could this happen with Marilyn and her parents?

I realized that the key to resolving this painful period was to try to induce Marilyn to come to Los Angeles and join her parents in a few family therapy sessions as a possible last resort to overcome their alienation. To their surprise Marilyn agreed and spent three emotionally laden sessions during one weekend. Listen to this early interaction between Marilyn and here parents.

"Marilyn," Grace began, "Ben and I have looked back at the time you were growing up and we both realize how we neglected you, though never deliberately. We were selfish and stupid and didn't realize how much you were suffering. We never looked closely at your life and tried to pretend you were happy and we were good parents. Now we know that just wasn't true."

"You never thought at all what was happening to me as a child," Marilyn shot back. "If you had even the slightest awareness of me, then it might have made a difference. Instead, I buried whatever I was feeling and never considered that you or Dad would want to hear my views on anything.

"My memory is filled with feeling alone and believing no one cared about me. I still often feel that way."

"No wonder you hated me," her mother replied sadly. "How could you have loved me for what I did to you, but I always loved you, even though I now know how much I neglected you."

"No, mother I didn't hate you. I hated myself."

"What do you mean?" Grace asked.

"I thought there was something wrong with me. For years I was afraid of facing people thinking they would see what was wrong with me. I sometimes thought I should just go away and hide; then maybe I'd be happy. No one would ever see me."

These and other memories had remained unspoken for many years causing untold grief and suffering that only now were being revived and reexamined. The forgotten experiences came to light revealing the intense emotions that had so colored their lives. Slowly this family healed as they came to understand that forgiveness from all of them was needed and to finally put these alienating reactions to rest.

I'm used to small miracles happening in therapy. People want to change and better their lives. It is natural for parents and children to want to share love and enjoy being together. Eliminating their suffering is the key to change and provides the impetus to pursue the reconciliation.

In our final session, Marilyn finally revealed why she was unable to accept reconciliation. With much crying and an inner pressure to finally resolve her plight Marilyn admitted that it wasn't the emptiness and aloneness and feeling so inferior and hate filled that had severely crippled her existence. Rather, she suffered inwardly believing that neither of her parents wanted her or loved her. She suffered believing there was something so terribly wrong with her that she could not be loved. And for much of her life she lived only partly alive. Living without love is a life without living. Listen to their words.

"Marilyn, my darling, I did love you. I never felt anything else. I'm so sorry for not showing you that love. I always thought you were wonderful. I can never forgive myself if you don't tell me that you can love me too. I need to hear you. I love you, please believe me. I love you more than my own life. Please believe me."

Marilyn sat, tears streaming down her face unable to move or to respond.

"Marilyn," I whispered, "believe it. Believe your mother. You've waited all your life for the love that is now there for you."

"No, No. No."

"Marilyn, just a tiny step and you can hold your mother and feel the love you've waited for. Marilyn, take it. You have suffered enough."

And Marilyn rose and went to her mother and continued to cry as though her heart would break. But I knew that finally the breaking of her heart had stopped. It was mending. Marilyn had taken her first step to overcome her anger and to fill the emptiness of her heart. She had accepted her mother's love and in the sharing of tears the healing had begun.

The remainder of the session was one of tenderness and forgiveness. Marilyn forgave both her parents for their neglect and essential abandonment of her. At my suggestion her parents forgave Marilyn for her withdrawal and anger that affected them so many years earlier and thereafter.

When Marilyn and her parents left my office, walking as a family, I sat for many minutes dwelling in my own inner world where love resided. How simple and yet so complex is the love that we all crave and need. Tears came to my eyes as I thought of how close these three people came to living in a world without the love that would now fill their lives.

Although the case of Ben and Grace came from my clinical practice most people can resolve problems without therapy. They can use a variety of techniques such as the ones I've introduced in this book to overcome conflicts and handicaps in their struggle to improve their lives.

I'd like to introduce you to an exercise that I call the "Inner Sanctuary." It is designed to allow you to overcome major conflicts that you might be carrying, which involve important people from your past and present life. The condition is frequently described as carrying "emotional baggage." The exercise gives you a way to forgive these significant persons for misunderstandings, poor parenting, rejections, anger and abuse.

The various emotions that often spring up between people often linger and remain imbedded within us continuing to negatively affect us, even to the point that they can be the most destructive elements in our personality. This exercise allows us to reexamine our inner world by creating a special room, temple or sanctuary, as such inner places are frequently called. Perhaps you have tried a similar exercise in the past. If so, I'd strongly encourage you to resume it. If not, then try to establish this inner place of peace and contentment where you will be meeting those with whom you wish to communicate.

Remember the objective is to call the person into your Inner Sanctuary to forgive him or her. You first will express the hurt that you carry, then how you may have contributed to the conflicts in the relationship, then ways to change your attitude and behavior and the same for your guest. You end by forgiving each other and expressing your renewed love. These experiences can be highly emotional and cleansing.

EXERCISE NO. 11: THE INNER SANCTUARY

Sit in a comfortable chair. Close your eyes. Take several deep breaths and feel your body relax. Now breathe normally. Visualize your entire body relaxing and feel tension draining from your mind, as well as your body. Now imagine that you are in a very special room. Some like a simple unembellished room. Others pick a chapel setting or a temple that conveys a spiritual quality. You can be sitting at a table or on a comfortable chair or even a throne. In general, the room is like a sanctuary filled with flowers and conveying a deep sense of tranquility and peace.

Now turn your attention inwardly, into your inner self. You are entering that place where you hold forgotten memories of all important persons from your past. You know that this is the time to face whatever issues have influenced your past relationships. You know that you will not hide from any conflicts that have affected you during your life. Once these conflicts are in the open, forgiveness will take place and it will end with acknowledging your love for each other.

You will now call out to one of these people. Let's start with your mother. Your mother appears in your sanctuary and sits near you. Or you can be walking in a garden and are joined by your mother. Your place of meeting is whatever you make it.

After welcoming your mother into your sanctuary, the dialogue will immediately ensue. It may become loud and angry. The dialogue contains feelings that you have harbored for years. You will face issues of anger, guilt and withdrawal. You will hear your voice and your mother's voice from the past and all the emotions that have remained buried. Voices that are now awakening. Believe in what you hear. It all comes from you. Be completely spontaneous. Do not censor your words or thoughts. This is an opportunity to truly learn about yourself and to make amends for pain you have carried for years. It is an opportunity to forgive your mother for what you believe she did to you and for you to seek forgiveness for what you may have brought into her life. This is an opportunity to revisit those memories and finally end the pain you carry.

Once the pain has been expressed you can tell your mother how you want to change and overcome your negative feelings. She can do likewise. You can tell her that you forgive her for what she did to you. Listen to your mother's response for she should also forgive you for creating so much unhappiness in her life, if indeed it happened that way. You end by saying to your mother that you love her. And your mother says that she loves you very much.

The following is an excerpt of a session from a patient, whom I'll call Josie, whose mother had died many years earlier. Although she spoke out loud, you may do it all internally or by speaking out loud. Try both ways and you can also alternate techniques. The people you call to you may be alive or dead. Either way their aliveness that you address is in you.

EXAMPLE NO. 1: From a 69 year-old woman.

"Mother, thank you for coming to visit me. I've waited for many years to gain the courage to talk to you. We have so much to say to each other; so much that we never talked about before. I want you to know that I love you. I'm sorry that I never told you after I had gone away."

Mother: "I've also waited to talk to you. You've been a bad child running away as soon as you could. You left me alone and I suffered enormously."

Josie: "Mother, I didn't call you here to complain but you may as well know that your suffering was nothing compared to what I felt. You never protected me when Dad screamed at me for things I never did. You always took Todd's side even though he always started our fights. You were drunk half the time and my friends made fun of you. You say you suffered. Imagine living with someone like you."

Mother: "None of that was my fault. It was the only way I could live with your father. He tormented me and beat me not just with words. Don't you remember my screaming for him to stop? He never cared that you and Todd were there. He'd beat me anyway...."

Josie: "I do remember all that. I'm sorry for how angry I would get at you. I was afraid of Dad and didn't know what to do."

After airing much pain from her childhood Josie and her mother took the first steps toward reconciling and forgiveness.

Josie: "Mother, I understand how you suffered and I wish now that your life would have been better. You deserved much better. I want you to know that I'm truly sorry for what I added to your misery and suffering."

Mother: "Josie, I don't know if I deserve your kind words. I see how much my behavior made you suffer and for that I'll never forgive myself."

Josie: "No mother. You need to forgive yourself. I want to forgive myself for being such a bad daughter to you for so long. I want you to know that I love you and I want us to feel loving toward each other."

Mother: "I love you too. I love you very much. I forgive everything that you ever did to me. I understand that as a child you had to do whatever you could to protect yourself since I didn't protect you."

EXAMPLE NO. 2: Told to me by a man, Norman, in his early 70's.

Norman: "Father, I called you to visit me. For many years I have felt much sorrow knowing that I had not been loving to you. I have wanted to reach out when you were alive but somehow could never do more than offer you a minimal degree of affection. I felt that you were displeased with me and judged me when I was small. I never told you how much you affected me and how much anger I held inside. I suffered with guilt and depression all the time. I feel terrible knowing how many times I wanted to hurt you and get even for what I believed was your rejection and scorn.

"I know now that you suffered enormously after your accident and felt badly you couldn't play with me or even go to my sports games or school conferences. I was angry that you just seemed to lock yourself in your room and never even talk to me. Only later did I understand how depressed you had become, but as a child I blamed you for my own misery. Dad, you suffered so much and it makes me sad knowing that I can never make up to you for my own avoidance and rejection of you."

Father: "Whatever happened and whatever you did I know it was not done out of malice or not loving me. I made your life very difficult by ignoring you. Please, forgive me, for all the suffering I caused you. Forgive me for not showing you more love and understanding."

Norman: "Dad, I do forgive you. When I think that you were never able to walk again and how much you hated the wheelchair I could cry. I finally just avoided you when you were suffering so much. I know you wanted me to be a great athlete as you had been, but I think I made you suffer by remaining mediocre. I suffered because I know I could have been much better.

"Dad, I want you to know that I apologize for my stupidity and rejecting you and want your forgiveness. I love you very much and I only wish you could return so we could have the loving relationship that I know we wanted."

Father: "Norman, I understanding your anguish and suffering. I feel so sad even as I accept your forgiveness, which really isn't necessary. I'm sorry that I was not more understanding and couldn't deal better with my own problems. I guess I blamed the world for my suffering. I fully understand your reactions. I know that you tried your best and as a child didn't have the resources you now have. I'm sorry that I didn't try to be a better dad. I share in the suffering that we both had during that period of your life. I forgive you for whatever you believed you did that added to my suffering. I love you for sharing your feelings toward me and forgiving me for all that happened. I love you very much."

When Norman finally overcame his inhibitions to face his older years and make this time of his life more satisfying and happy, he was able to face his past. He had suffered with enormous guilt all his life and was unable to find peace and joy in his existence. He found much use of his sanctuary calling to it countless people, including his mother, three siblings, cousins, two wives, his children and many friends.

It is not only the deceased that you can call to face you. It can be anybody with whom you share love and/or conflicts. The sanctuary is merely a device to look within you. Many people can do it without the formality of a sanctuary. In my experience, however, this device helps bring forth ideas, feelings and memories that are often elusive otherwise. The perceived safety of the sanctuary gives aliveness to your recollections from your past. Much resolution and much unexpressed feelings, that include love, are revealed there. The catharsis of forgiveness and the expression of love within the sanctuary of your mind are very healing.

The episodes I briefly described were filled with much crying, anger, guilt and pain over the continuing suffering as patients relived the blame heaped on their parents and themselves. Finally, mutual forgiveness and the expression of love brought an end to the suffering. It gives you an idea of what such meetings can accomplish. The tenor of the meetings and what came forth are fairly typical when you are seeking ways to forgive.

Many meetings are filled only with love and the recall of memories of happiness and sharing special experience. This exercise is to show you a way to resolve problems that have caused you suffering, but many significant people you call to your inner sanctuary will bring forth joy alone.

In a future chapter on creativity we will take this technique another step and discuss ways to meet with people you do not personally know. Why not call forth a great artist or writer? How about a discussion with Einstein or Darwin? All the voices obviously reflect you. But you will be very surprised at the dialogue that ensues. You can ask these people for advice and suggestions on improving your life. Don't believe that because the voices and words are part of yourself that you will know all the answers. Many things come up when formulated this way that will surprise and may even shock you. Later, when we discuss creativity you will find how this kind of dialogue can assist you toward realizing your dreams of a more fruitful life.

REFLECTIONS

Love is a source of wondrous feelings that nurture our souls. Yet it is so easy to feel unloved, alone and abandoned. Rejection with its feelings of deprivation may occur inadvertently without deliberate intent caused by anger and hate.

Children are not born with love in their hearts. Their love evolves from interaction with their caretakers. They are responders and reflectors of what is given to them. When loved they respond with love. When rejected they respond with anger or hurt, or a feeling of worthlessness and a belief that the world is unloving.

Some children fare well with a minimum of interaction and love. Others crave and need enormous amounts of affection and devotion without which they may respond with anger and hurt and withdraw into a reclusive existence or anti-social behavior.

A child doesn't know how to evaluate the absence of love or parents who occasionally withdraw into their own suffering and for a period of time stop showing love. Children react to what they perceive and imagine. Unless something radically changes in their life they carry the doubt of their lovability with them and sometimes pass it to their children. But above all it prevents them from living in peace and inner happiness.

In our later years the absence of love becomes increasingly disturbing. We look for ways to forgive those we resented and those who roused anger. We look for ways to recover and resurrect love that had faded away. We try to awaken dormant love with new relationships. We try to return to our past and reengage old friends and even acquaintances. We turn again to our parents, even when they have long died. We need to forgive and to believe that we are loved.

Ben and Grace finally found the family they never had. Beth would become the star of this new family and know genuine love from her grandparents. Marilyn would require time to adjust to the love offered her and time to share her own awakening love with her parents. Each had learned that holding on to the past and continuing to live out memories of suffering and regrets had prevented them from finding the love and peace they so desperately wanted.

> *Living for now, in the NOW, is essential for truly coming alive. Although this is valid throughout life, it is especially important when people reach retirement. There is no better time for people to reach out to the love that is within their grasp. Love comes from friends, animals and acquaintances, in addition to the love of a child, grandchild or from someone who shares your life.*

Many older people no longer have a life partner for love. Many do not have children or grandchildren. What of them? They, too, have many resources for love that will provide fulfillment. The wisdom and knowledge that people have accumulated throughout life will guide them toward activities that will suit them. Consider the following ways to discover new venues to experience love that could provide greater meaning in your life.

- Sharing knowledge and experiences with special friends.
- Bringing a dog, cat or bird into your life.
- Acting as a confidante to younger people.
- Becoming a Big Brother and Big Sister for young children.
- Finding ways to give to those in need and actively participating in their lives.
- Reading to the blind, helping to nurture the ill.
- Finding like-minded people who provide support for many charities.
- Becoming an active environmentalist and sharing the love of nature with others.
- Forming close relationships with the children of friends or other family members.
- Nurturing your own inner resources to love yourself.
- Becoming immersed in music and falling in love with the beauty of visual artists.
- Turning to studies that elevate your spirit and becoming part of a group that seeks similar development.
- Exploring religion and finding love in a Supreme Being.

Taking one or more of the many paths to finding love will amply reward you. This is the time to shed all hesitation, overcome all mixed feelings, and go forward. The vicissitudes of love are boundless. We need to feel loved and to give love to make our last years fulfilling and vital. Love is out there. Seek it.

CONCLUSIONS

The bonds of the mother, father and child are like no other. Inherent in most creatures in the world, and most complex with humans, bonds can never be undone. Yet many dangers exist to diminish and even to destroy that tie and the underlying love that nurtures it. Even the awareness of such dangers does not necessarily curtail their presence. Anger in any form frightens the child; arguments between the parents evoke insecurity; jealousy of siblings may arouse parental punishment; abuse destroys trust and over-control prevents needed independence. Threats and actual abandonment infringe on a child's integrity and sense of safety. Their identity as a secure and loving person is scarred leaving them vulnerable to troubled relationships.

When children grow up, barriers are sometimes erected to protect whatever sense of self remains. They close out the pain and deny the bond with parents. By denying their love they exist in a shadowy world determined by their underlying need to be loved and the fear of reaching for it. Children can't make the determination of how they are raised and even parents are often the victim of circumstances beyond their control. Adults, however, especially as they get older, are uniquely ready to break through the barriers that otherwise might determine their future family connections. There should be no doubt about taking whatever steps are needed to change impoverished relationships within family units.

Chapter Eight

THE PATH TO SPIRITUALITY

He enjoys true leisure who has time to improve his soul's estate.

— H. D. Thoreau

Prophets of Nature, we to them will speak
A lasting inspiration, sanctified
By reason, blest by faith: what we have loved,
Others will love, and we will teach them how;
Instruct them how the mind of man becomes
A thousand times more beautiful than the earth
On which he dwells.

—William Wordsworth

Perhaps next to finding love, those who enter retirement seek ways to find or to enhance their spirituality. Through religion, meditation, communing with nature, reading great books and inhaling the mystical words of great poets, people discover paths to spirituality. Many believe that the presence of an inner spiritual instinct carries them into a higher plane of existence, a kind of mystical or otherworldly sense of self.

Some people feel they always exist in that special state of mind while others feel that they are transported there only under certain circumstances. It may come walking along a seaside cliff and watching a magical sunset. Being among trees hidden from the cacophony of city noise or being at home listening to music you love may lead to a transcendent experience. Occasionally just being alone with yourself while in a calm and reflective state, perhaps while meditating, can lead to a transitory state of transcendence. Being in church or temple sharing a meaningful sermon or hearing the stirring voices of the choir may take you into another realm of being.

Spirituality is the great equalizer. The belief in an innate spiritual self is widely held by most religions and ethnic groups. As long as man has felt awe in the wonder and beauty of nature he has been conscious of a special inner feeling that connects him to the universe.

Spirituality is abstract and thus can't be easily defined. However, it creates a deep sense of self and is likened to love. Many people believe that love for children and grandchildren is part of the feeling of spirituality. Offering alms, giving to charity, assisting people in need, believing in God and prayer are components of spirituality. Perhaps the closest one can come to spirituality is a deep internal feeling that appears at times that transports a person into another realm of consciousness. Some call it transcendence that may occur during mystical experiences, creative moments, reacting with awe to nature's magnificence and as part of being religious.

Many patients come to see me wanting to achieve a more spiritually fulfilling life. Charlene, 64, entered therapy seeking to overcome a feeling of emptiness. To her, life had become meaningless. She believed it was due to her inability to feel spiritual or to believe in God. Seeking spirituality was equated with finding herself.

Charlene had regularly attended church for many years but admitted that she was confused about her feelings toward God. Over the years she had tried different churches but it made no difference.

"Doctor, I'm a nothing person. I can't feel the presence of God or any spirit inside me. But I know I'm a good person. I give to charity and help people whenever I can.

But I don't feel anything. I've always wanted to be a spiritual person and believe in God. I pray a lot, mainly for other people. I pray for the sick and the homeless and for the dying. But, no matter how much I try, nothing changes. I'm dying inside."

"Are you able to have any feelings about anything?" I gently asked.

"Of course," she replied, surprised at my question. "I love my husband and my two children and four grandchildren. I love my friends. Those are not the feelings I lack."

"Can you describe more specifically what you do lack?"

"Feelings of the spirit. Feelings from God. I believe in God and pray, but I feel nothing. I listen to music and walk among the trees and admire them but I don't experience a deep connection. I'm lacking a sense of spirituality.

"I know that I should love beautiful things and music and sometimes I believe that I do. But when I'm truly honest with myself I know that I pretend so I won't become desolate. I sometimes don't think I know myself. Like I'm lacking any insight into who I am. Like there's a cover over my soul."

Charlene's perplexing lack of spirituality is actually quite common though not always expressed so vividly. Most people don't really think about whether they're spiritual or not. If spirituality is meaningful to them, then whatever they feel in that regard is accepted as normal. Spiritual connections can occur in so many ways outside of religion that some aspect of it is generally experienced.

Charlene's search for meaning became strongly tied to her need to find her spiritual self. In an intellectual sense she believed in God but lacking an emotional spiritual experience she felt a deep emptiness in life.

"It's important that I don't spend my last years on earth unable to connect to spirituality," Charlene stated. "I want to feel there's a greater purpose and meaning in life. I think it's connected to my soul and I must put to rest any concern that I have no soul. I know that our souls go on forever and having a soul must mean that I have spirit inside me. I need to believe and feel it."

Charlene's fear of not being spiritual became connected to having a soul and her belief in an afterlife. Her quandary was never truly believing in God and the immortality of her soul.

> As people get older the purpose of living changes and they need to know more about their existence. As the end of their life approaches they need to come to an understanding of their place in this world. They feel more strongly that much in life can't be explained through reason and logic. Many believe through faith. Others believe by experiencing a deep sense of fullness and joy. Our spirituality is a matter of becoming free to experience this inner feeling.

Whether the feeling is mystical or a newfound love or being filled with a sense of nature's beauty or believing in your prayers makes no difference. The presence of spirituality is determined by the quality of the feeling that is not detected by our usual five senses. Spirituality comes to us through another intrinsic part of our inner world. Words are woefully lacking in describing what is felt. Perhaps this is one time when you might say that when it happens you'll know it.

"Charlene, there are many who do not feel spiritual but never question it. Instead they feel empty and depressed and often question their ability to love. Seeking spirituality is often directionless since its very nature is not specifically connected to external actions. Otherwise merely going to church and praying or giving alms might be conceived as spiritual. For many it is, but only because their sense of spirituality exists independent of those actions. Rather, I believe that spirituality is connected to the love of others and to self-love."

"Yes," she murmured. "I feel that is true for me."

With an intense need to rid herself of inner demons and unacceptable feelings Charlene told of her impoverished childhood. Ignored by her mother, a frightened and passive

woman, severely criticized by her gruff and abusive father
and intimidated and taunted by her two siblings, an older
brother and a younger sister, Charlene grew up feeling
alone and unloved. Her fantasies involved much anger and
destructiveness against all members of her family. She
deeply envied the love she believed her family shared that
excluded her.

When she finally left home she had created a façade of
being loving and kind, but inwardly maintained a deep envy
of everyone who she felt had more than she. Guilt and a
feeling of unworthiness gripped her, especially when others
offered her love and kindness.

Charlene, at a loss to know how to overcome her envy,
begged for a solution. In addition to her continuing therapy
I introduced two Imagery exercises to help her. To develop
the Imagery I asked her, "What do you need to do to begin
to feel loving and spiritual?"

"Whatever I do, I'll only be pretending," she replied.

"No," I reassured her. "You will find ways to overcome
your envy even as you find ways to love others and yourself
in your real life. Try to go inside yourself and discover what
you need to make that happen."

The following two imagery exercises that came from
Charlene's therapy can be practiced by others who may be
facing a similar problem. The exercises are an adjunct to
the steps that Charlene took to change. They are the kinds
of Imagery that will increase positive feelings and self-
regard.

EXERCISE NO. 12: SAYING GOOD-BYE TO ENVY

Go into a state of relaxation. Imagine that you
are visualizing your inner self and you see a
large completely unsavory mass of unknown
tissue, and know it is your envious self. It
reaches into every part of your body and into
your brain and mind. You see it as smothering
all other feelings and that it is slowly
destroying you. In a thunderous voice say that
you hate that part of yourself and you will no
longer keep it inside you. With deep conviction

and through the power of your mind you order all envious parts of you to disappear forever.

In a blinding flash of light your body becomes completely free of the insidious mass and you become light, free, loving and in a state of near ecstasy. You have conquered your envy and say to your self proudly and convincingly that you will never feel envy toward anyone again.

EXERCISE NO. 13: BECOMING SPIRITUAL

Continue your state of relaxation. This is an end-state Imagery exercise.

Imagine yourself as a totally loving and fulfilled person. See yourself reaching out with love to your children, grandchildren, friends, strangers and to God. People respond to you by giving you love and warmth and exclaim how wonderful a person you are. You feel joyful and brimming with goodness. You smile as you realize that you are at complete peace with yourself and the world. You feel joyful and brimming with goodness as you realize that you are at complete peace with yourself and the world. You feel connected to nature, spirit and self. You finally look up at the sky and bless yourself for having become a loving and spiritual person.

"I'll practice the imagery," Charlene said softly. "I really want to get rid of feeling so envious. I hate myself when I feel that way. What else can I do?"

"Let's find out," I responded. "Do you have any doubt in your mind that you love your children and grandchildren?"

For a moment Charlene hesitated. "Of course, I don't. For a second I even began to wonder if that were true. I don't want to end up doubting myself. I know that I love them."

"There's no doubt in your mind about that?" I asked cautiously.

Again Charlene hesitated. "I don't think so but now I'm not so sure. Can I be such a fake that I don't even love my children and husband?"

"Charlene, there are gradations of people's ability to love, but to be faithful to yourself it must be genuine. You will know the difference provided you don't hide from anything that's interfering with believing it. I believe that you genuinely love your children and grandchildren. This is one area that is rarely doubted.

"You know then that you have the ability to love. You need to extend that belief. You have to give love to others even when you're not certain it's genuine. If necessary you pretend until you reach that point where the pleasure in giving and loving seems natural. You will enjoy being loving, not only because of a feeling inside you but from the responses you will get from others. Loving people get love back in spades. When you give unselfishly what returns is genuine love. You will feel it and thrive on it."

Slowly Charlene turned her attention to the other areas where she was uncertain of her love. She had pretended to be religious. She had lied to people to make them see her as good and loving.

She quickly learned that though pretending is useful as a learning tool it must be seen strictly as a tool and not as your specific way of relating to the world.

Charlene came to the point where she had admitted to herself and to me all the ways her life style interfered with becoming spiritual. Her envy gradually diminished and her pretense was no longer needed.

She forgave her parents and siblings for abuses from her past and acknowledged to them how she had hurt them. Much soul-searching occurred and it started her true path toward spirituality. She learned that forgiveness is a sign of a spiritual person. Holding in anger and hate is counter-love and counter-spiritual.

"Do I have to become more religious?" she asked one day.

"That is entirely up to you. Many people believe that spirituality is closely linked to formal religion. Others feel it's separate. Since you're already religious you can observe your interaction with it and decide how much it will contribute to becoming spiritual."

"I want to do everything possible to change my life."

"You can do it. Becoming spiritual is becoming a whole person, a loving and giving and nurturing person. I believe that you already have the feelings necessary to achieve what you want. It's a matter of becoming free to experience who you are."

When Charlene asked for specific suggestions to help her become spiritual I responded with words that would be accurate for all seekers of spirituality.

"Just follow your inclinations and remain flexible," I said. "If you try to become spiritual you'll get bogged down in rituals or behavior that only fit your idea of what spirituality is and that may be very limiting. It's much better to be guided by love, sharing yourself, curiosity, seeking new friends, and activities. You will eventually know your state of mind."

Some experiences that Charlene described to me showed the way she had taken to become loving. She told me about finding a butterfly lying on the sidewalk that appeared to be dying. She picked it up and placed in a bed of flowers. She placed leaves around it to protect it. She believed that the butterfly stared at her thankfully. "I know that it was quite unlikely," she said, "but I felt a connection with it, nevertheless."

Each visit I heard of new experiences, new friends and new deeds. She began to feel the desire to devote more time to her religion and decided to visit a number of churches and meet the ministers. She finally settled on a new church after being stirred by several sermons and succumbing to the angel-like singing of its choir. "My heart was filled with a sense of the sublime after hearing the music," she said. "It somehow made me believe more strongly in God and Heaven. Can music give you an exalted sense of faith?" she pondered.

"Many things lead to a growing belief in God," I replied. "Perhaps of all the arts music is our closest realization of God's power on earth."

At the urging of an old friend she became an active sponsor of a charity that provided funds for research for children's cancer. Among the various activities were included visiting and writing letters to children dying of cancer. She told me how difficult it was seeing the brave children and how she had to fight desperately to avoid crying in their presence. Instead she became sought after by doctors and social workers to talk to particularly sad and frightened children. She became known for her sensitivity and the love that flowed from her.

She and her husband spent a weekend at a retreat in the mountains above Malibu. She said that the quietness and the long periods of silence practiced by the weekend participants brought her closer to her inner thoughts and the beauty that resided within her.

She learned to meditate and decided to make it part of her daily life. She offered her services to read two hours a week to the blind and an afternoon selling flowers in a concession in one of the local hospitals.

The time had come when I knew that Charlene no longer needed to see me. For almost five months she had worked diligently to find a new path in life. Initially it started as a search for spirituality. But it was the path of love that she followed. She did not question becoming spiritual or mystical. Instead she followed her inclinations and reached out to others and to meaningful activities. She gave unstintingly to charities, the ill, small children, animals and to preserving nature.

She no longer asked whether she was becoming spiritual. There was no longer any need to do so. Once you feel an inner spirit, an inner belief in God and especially knowing that you are loved and give love freely to others the presence of an inner spirit is taken for granted.

One day as our work together was nearing its end I said, "Participating in church is special to you and although you only mentioned it once I know that you pray and believe your prayers are heard. Do I have to say that you have achieved what you had come here for?"

"No," she replied softly. "I no longer question my spirituality because I live with love and freedom. I take for granted that I'm a spiritual person. I feel there's a divine light inside me and it's expressed in my love. Whatever others feel toward me I accept, much as I accept my love toward them.

When we said goodbye to each other we both had tears in our eyes. Charlene had learned the power of love and I had learned once again of the intrinsic goodness of people and how self-growth is always possible when motivation and persistence exist. Charlene had found a new world that gave her inner love and peace. As much as she brought love into the lives of so many, she was also filled with the love and caring given to her by countless people. Charlene had truly found the divine light that filled her soul. She had achieved the inner spirituality that she had sought. Spirituality nurtured by her love.

REFLECTIONS

Charlene began the path toward spirituality, hopeful and motivated. She quickly found the ways to move into a new world of love and friendship that had eluded her for years. She no longer thought of herself as handicapped or unable to love. Rather she came to understand that her upbringing had interfered with her normal growth and her intrinsic spirituality had been stymied, but not eradicated. Her desire to become spiritual became the power that guided her toward overcoming her handicap.

No matter what initial handicaps that people have, everyone has the potential of reaching a spiritual and loving way. The paths that we take are personal and reflect who we are. There are as many ways of becoming spiritual as there are people.

One may be motivated to seek freedom from hate, envy, greed, jealousy, doubt and obsessive preoccupations. As a person progresses toward a spiritual existence, obstacles fall away. A fully realized spiritual self becomes the objective.

Spirituality is not measured in quantity, but in the quality of your existence. It doesn't depend on complete freedom, but on the direction and purpose of your life. Little things become important. The hug you give a friend, the charity you show toward the needy, the love you feel toward others and yourself are all components of a spiritual existence.

Some people become mystical and study to learn more of the esoteric elements in life. Seeking God and praying for his support and guidance are part of spirituality for many. Creating something new, beautiful or useful can be spiritual. Identification with nature and helping to protect the beauty that surrounds us can be part of a spiritual life.

Above all is the feeling of love. Love takes many forms and all are connected to spirituality. Love that comes with sharing your life and worldly goods. Love that is freely given and felt toward family and friends. Love that is felt toward animals, nature and our planet. Love that is felt for yourself.

For countless years the connection of religion and spirituality has existed, but has often been subjected to questioning. Is spirituality a condition of being religious or is it more dependent on an inner essence that we all have independent of religion? Certainly, religion can be and generally is a major stimulus for people seeking to become spiritual. But it is not the only way and in itself doesn't guarantee that a person will become spiritual.

Rather an inner sense of self, a feeling of wholeness and a connection to God that may not involve formal religion become representative of spirituality. It may include the soul's connection to the world and God. The question is often asked, "Can one be spiritual without a belief in God? Or does being spiritual mean a belief in God?"

Many believe that spirituality requires a belief in the immortality of the soul, and its ultimate destination to join God. Thus we have an inner spirit that elevates and transports us and is expressed as a belief in the transcendence of the spirit. The acceptance of reincarnation frequently accompanies this belief.

For many people the first inclination of questioning their spirituality occurs during a serious illness or facing the death of a loved one or themselves. The fear of death and the unknown spurs people to reexamine their lives leading to the arousal of spirituality. As one gets older friends die and illness becomes more frequent. Retirement provides the matrix when such questions arise.

As already noted, spirituality can occur under numerous circumstances, belief systems, and ideologies. It comes in many forms and thus is experienced differently by different people. For some it may be constantly present. For others it may appear sporadically and in different guises. For many, spirituality involves joy, hope, love and mysticism. Sometimes a moment of deep passion awakens spiritual feelings. Whatever the stimulus the inner change is easily recognized. Such a feeling energizes and arouses senses that otherwise may not occur.

> *Spirituality is based on our existence and our relationship to self, the world and the universe. It provides us with insight and meaning. Spirituality is experienced as an integrative force that makes us feel whole and connected to the outside world. It is the link to our true essence and to our total self.*

CONCLUSIONS

Spirituality comes with the opening of your mind to the goodness within. It is boundless and comes in many guises. Spirituality cloaks the art of living and lightens the soul and the steps you take. It can't be defined, but it can be felt. Be genuinely giving and loving. Remove anger and envy from your heart. You will find spirituality. It is within you and only needs to be freed of doubts and restraints. You will know when you have found it.

Spirituality is the poetry of the soul.

Chapter Nine

CREATIVITY FOR SENIORS

Imagination is everything. It is the preview of life's coming attractions.

—Albert Einstein

Without this playing with fantasy no creative work has ever yet come to birth. The debt we owe to the play of the imagination is incalculable.

— Carl Jung

Don't be afraid of the space between your dreams and reality. If you can dream it, you can make it so.

— Belva Davis

You are a creative person. You are filled with a sparkling imagination. You are entering a unique world where new vistas and new opportunities await. Becoming older has many advantages and developing your creativity stands in the foreground. Creativity blends the energies of inventiveness, exploration, spirituality and personal growth.

The world is replete with artists, writers, scientists, inventors, teachers and people from all walks of life, who reached their highest level of creativity in their senior years. Obstacles and barriers were swept aside as they remained fully immersed in their creativity and continuing productiveness.

Because of a widespread myth that creativity is for the young, many seniors ignore the potential for developing their creativity. You, however, will not be caught up in denying this potential. Whether you are 60 or 90 or even 100 you will unhesitatingly move into the beckoning arena of creativity. It is imperative that you believe in the potential that lies within you as a senior. And you must work hard at realizing these opportunities to increase your mental power and enhance your imagination. Dr. Gene Cohen, Director of the Center on Aging, Health & Humanities and Professor of Health Care and Psychiatry at George Washington University, prophetically wrote a book about retirement titled "The Creative Age."

Becoming older offers an unparalleled opportunity to reconnect with your creative self. Think back to your childhood. Remember building toys from everyday objects and playing games that took you and friends to an unknown world. You created imaginary playmates, built castles in the sky, believed in magic, talked to spirits, ghosts and magical people. You didn't try to eliminate such unrealistic games or playmates. Instead you welcomed them into your life.

Painting a picture was another vehicle to an imaginary world. Whether you attempted to reproduce a real object on canvas or merely painted whatever feelings guided you, your painting represented your creative self. If you only painted smudges or smeared globs of paint on paper or just piled random colors on a canvas you knew what they meant. The outsider, even Mom, could only guess what the abstract painting represented. But you could describe what each segment meant. Nothing was meaningless. Your mind was your playground and using it was natural. And it all remains waiting to be rekindled. It only takes stirring your imagination and learning ways to bring it back to life.

Childhood has been gone for years and it is possible that your creative drive might have lessened. But the creative instincts and interests never fully disappear. Even if seemingly gone, I can assure you that they're not. Many adults do not recall their creative childhood, but it's there.

Scarcely a day goes by without your imagination revealing itself. Night dreams and day dreams abound. Fantasies color your existence. When you imagine or reflect on some current or future activity you are using your creative imagination. Taking over the role of a favorite athlete or artist or picturing yourself in a story that you are reading is a sign of your continuing creativity. Imagining how you would handle a political situation or being the advisor to a famous person is another form of creativity. And if you dream of being that politician or athlete or artist, such dreams are made of the stuff of creativity.

Awakening the Creative Drive

Even if your creative self was never encouraged during your childhood, don't despair. The creative drive is merely lying dormant and only needs to be nudged and awakened. By the time you finish this chapter you will know countless ways to stimulate your creative juices and overcome blocks to creativity. You will be ready to bring forth something unique, something that is strictly a reflection of you. You will learn a variety of special techniques and tools to help you become whatever you want. You won't be limited by a narrow area of the creative spectrum. You will have the knowledge to develop your creativity in any area that you choose.

Many people try a variety of creative outlets searching for the most satisfying and exciting activity to fill their time. Why not paint a picture or carve a sculpture? How about writing a poem or essay and why not try your hand at a novel? Creatively abounds in the way you interact with people, how you show love and engage in sparkling conversations. Creativity may appear in the way you cook or garden and even in the way you enjoy solitude. How does creativity fit into those areas you wonder? Read on.

Can an older person become creative strictly by will? The short answer is YES. If you are willing to learn techniques and methods leading to its fulfillment, you will become a creative person. Your age has nothing to do with it. It's your desire, wish, motivation and persistent efforts that are your touchstones.

Are there any restraints or restrictions to expressing creativity? The answer is NO. We all have inherent creative drives. The mind and brain are like muscles. They need to be exercised and trained and carefully nurtured and they will perform. You can depend on it.

Becoming a Believer in your Ability to Change your Life

You must become a believer in your ability to change your life and put creativity at its center. So what can you do to make it happen?

- First, it is important to recognize whether you carry any conscious negative beliefs about your creative self. Some people doubt that they can be creative or believe they lack something called talent or genius. Talent is not the decisive force in creativity and generally can't be taught, but that is not true of creativity. Creativity can be taught and augmented. Many discoveries, artistic projects, inventions, visual arts, all forms of writing and other original activities come from the process of utilizing your creative imagination. It is independent of talent or that inherent ability that makes one naturally an artist, musician or writer.

- Second, having an inherent gift to draw as a child does not predict that child will become an artist. Rather studying art, learning to draw and understanding the use of color plus a strong desire to become an artist become the forces behind the realization of an artist's dream. By understanding methods and learning techniques you can become creative or enhance your creativity. You need to believe in your ability to produce something worthwhile.

- Third, look into your previous attitudes regarding your creative interests and attempts. Were they ignored by parents or teachers? Did your parents emphasize excelling in school or in sports? Was your free-wheeling creative energy diverted or suppressed? Childhood creativity is often ignored or misunderstood as a powerful force and thus insufficient emphasis is placed on it.

- Fourth, do you have any mental or emotional barriers that need to be removed? If you believe that you cannot produce something worthwhile, it is not too likely you would spend time painting a picture or writing a book. So you need to extricate yourself from any negativity. Do you believe that you're too old to learn new tricks? I can assure you, once again, that you are not too old unless you believe it.

By following the ways to retain youthfulness that fill the pages of this book, you will feel younger and more vital. You will believe in your ability to think and act like a younger person. You will finally put to rest the mistaken idea that your age is determined by a calendar. Many people in their 80's and 90's are as young in spirit, mind and body as someone half their age. Becoming creative is clearly linked with the belief that you are young and vibrant, as well as being a believer in your ability to be creative.

Becoming creative is a personal and solo experience. Comparing yourself to anyone is not part of the process. We're all unique and different and will express our creative urges in individual ways.

Finally, you have arrived at the phase of life when you can truly realize a self you may have only dreamed about. You do not have to make your mark or earn a living from this endeavor or even gain the accolades of others. Even though others may benefit and appreciate whatever you produce, this is for you.

The Development of your Creativity

You will experience the development of your creativity as very positive and uplifting. Of the wide range of creative projects available, you must never view your efforts as frivolous or useless. You will not only enjoy your burgeoning creative self, you can have a ball with it. As you march through the second half of life, the opportunities for creativity are enormous.

Becoming a unique and exciting person is in your future. No more rote or uninteresting learning; everything will come out of your own desire to be distinctive and creative. The wonders of your imagination will guide you in your pursuit of the creative life. You have gained wisdom and maturity as an older adult that will facilitate your adopting new methods and procedures. You don't stop being logical and rational or avoid the rules or the needed techniques for any art. You will learn techniques that creative people have always used and some that are not so widely known but that I have found very useful for stimulating creativity.

> *As you cultivate your creative potential you will find a new power that will guide you and enhance your ability to become the vital and exciting person of your dreams.*

You will venture into many different areas, discovering that you are adventurous and daring. You will learn to create characters inside yourself that will help you write stories. You will have the same fervor and glee as a child when you paint. Your inner child is creative and puts up no obstacles. Imagine yourself in the mind of a child experiencing the newness of your thoughts and the sense of growing power that will sweep over you. Imagine it! Then become that child. Does all this sound impossible or pie in the sky? It isn't. Not only will you become more creative but you will want to jump with joy at your newfound freedom.

Experiencing Creativity

Pick up a paintbrush and paint without thought. Dig your hands into soft clay and mold a head or a turtle or something abstract. Buy a guitar or banjo and learn to play it. Then improvise and make up your own songs. Write poems to those you love and send them off. Write anything. Start an article, a short story. And how about a novel? Is any of this possible? Absolutely. You'll be surprised at how creative you are. You only have to give yourself a chance.

Perhaps nothing in this period of life will be as satisfying as creating something new. You don't have to indulge in creativity as an all day pursuit, although some of you might prefer that. The excitement of feeling something new and different brewing inside you and watching it spring forth is a peak moment in life. You can have many of them.

The ways are almost unlimited. You can design and plant a beautiful garden and watch your own flowers and vegetables grow. Being a part of nature's beauty and bounty is especially meaningful to people. Eating the food you grow is a special taste treat. Having an endless supply of your own flowers to cut and bring into your home is a unique gift to yourself.

There's creativity in the way you interact with people, especially with those you love. Make the relationship more alive by avoiding the clichés and mundane activities that often occupy our time. You will be surprised at what comes out. Play games with each other. You can do it with song, poetry and paintings. Intuition and empathy will begin to play a greater role in your relationships. You'll find wit, kidding around and intimate repartee adding zest and excitement to your interaction with friends and family. Creativity can be a shared experience as well as a singular one.

Believe in your ability to be creative. The potential is in you. Through your own efforts and desire you can make it happen. Creativity comes out of your own inner world. No one except you can make it happen. Sometimes we have blocks that seem to scuttle our creative urges. Such blocks can be removed. You can do it yourself. You will learn many techniques to do it. Here are a few ideas for starters.

Overcoming Creative Blocks

Never sit for more than a few minutes before a blank screen on your computer if you're trying to write or remain inactive when you desire to paint. Get up, stretch, go for a short walk, sing, and tell yourself repeatedly that when you return to your computer or easel the words or paint will flow. If they don't, get up again and go for a longer walk.

Place all your creativity under the control of your imagination. See yourself as a painter, a writer, a poet. Imagine yourself engaged in delightful and witty conversations. Write words that appear in your mind, even nonsense and meaningless thoughts. Laugh at your special humor and cry when you conceive something sad. Be immersed in your inner world. It will reward you.

Put yourself in the shoes of creative people you admire. Pretend you are someone you want to be. Then act to emulate and become like that person. Read their words out loud and act the part. Pour your creativity into your actions. You may discover a new you. The ways are unlimited. It's a new way to make yourself into an unlimited person. Is it possible? Try it. What can you lose?

All people are inherently creative. You are now learning ways to stimulate your creativity so it becomes an active part of your life. Creativity comes in different forms and goes far beyond the visual and auditory arts. It exists in the pursuit of spirituality, finding meaning in life, modifying thinking and belief systems, and improving athletic prowess.

Discovering ways to change behavior and mindsets can be highly creative. You can improve relationships and enhance intimacy by using imagination and creative intelligence. By being fluid and open to new ideas even dialogue can be creative and result in lively and free-wheeling conversations.

Once you learn the techniques to develop your creativity you'll recognize your uniqueness and know that you're not in competition with anyone. By enjoying your new skills you'll be able to overcome any inferiority, self doubts or fears that you will be unable to create anything meaningful. You will not compare your work with others. You will not react negatively when a person shows more skills or even more imagination, since they are strictly variations in the grand scheme of creativity.

You don't have to be perfect. An artist can paint and sculpt without having skills to make their art look realistic. Differences between classically trained artists and self-taught and folk artists can be marked but has little to do with creativity or quality.

Seniors are especially ready to develop into creative people, yet many doubt that they can produce anything of value. Therefore you need to eliminate your perceived sense of value in comparison to others, especially recognized artists, in order to minimize its impact on your work.

Anything produced is valuable as an expression of one's inner self and the ability to give birth to a special object. Some seniors will discover a new talent or revive a long buried talent. Some will have to overcome inhibitions that were set in motion in their childhood. Although much of creativity is a solo experience it can be a great way to become involved with new friends, groups and share the experience as well as having a new social world to enter. Having activities in common opens doors to friendships.

Creativity can be tied to self-awareness and self-knowledge, as well as to spiritual development. It can appear in how a person relates to nature, world conditions and polities. It involves thinking outside the box and the willingness to become a self-contained thinker and a readiness to stand up for one's beliefs.

> *Developing enthusiasm and joy in being creative is important. Creativity is tied to the freedom of the spirit, making a connection with a power that sometimes seems to be outside the self. Yet realizing that power comes from within is the source of your greatest strength. We are nurtured by our creative spirit.*

You are the creator. You are therefore the director of your own drama, the drama of changing yourself and making your dreams real. Since creativity is an action that takes place in the brain there are actual brain changes that enlarge one's capacity for thinking. Creativity is brain enhancement. It is exciting to imagine the growth of your brain. It is exciting to travel this new path toward a new you.

Creativity has intrigued writers for centuries and countless writers have tried to explain or theorize about the creative process. In 1926, Graham Wallas in his book *Art of Thought* simply and meaningfully described the process. He divided creativity into four phases: Preparation, Incubation, Illumination, Verification.

The Four Phases of Creativity

PREPARATION

The easiest phase to understand. It's a continuation of what you have been doing all your life—learning and acquiring information and knowledge. In the singular effort to be creative you merely focus on what interests you. Acquire as much knowledge as possible or as much as you believe you need to know. If you're trying to change a recognized scientific theory you will need vast amounts of information about what is known about the subject. If you want to paint a picture in a certain style you should study artists who paint in that style. However, if you paint in your own style then just go for it.

Fact-gathering intensifies when a specific interest kindles your imagination. Since it's not too likely that you will be focusing on developing a new complex theory of planetary motion your preparatory phase could be relatively brief. However, do whatever is needed to acquire information. Several older patients, one who was 79, returned to full time college to acquire the knowledge needed to pursue special interests.

If you want to learn to paint, your level of preparation might only entail learning about colors, various media, brushes and types of painting surfaces. A single beginner's class in art is probably all you need to start. However, it's worth noting that many artists of all ages started to draw and paint by merely getting some paint, a few brushes, a couple of canvases and starting. You can either try to copy a still life, another painting or attack the canvas armed only with abandonment and a lively imagination. Just do it.

If you desire more advanced painting techniques and styles join a class or get private instruction. Art classes can be particularly enjoyable as you share your new experiences with others and perhaps make new friends. If your interest evolves you might enjoy taking some classes in art history or make art galleries openings and tours part of your outside activities. This can lead to another world of ideas and gives you a greater understanding of the changes in art and society over the centuries.

To sum up:

The **Preparatory** phase is an information and reflective period that provides the inner resources needed to be creative. The more you learn the more likely you'll reach your goal. Normal education and the imagination provide much of the information needed for your creativity. All creators prepare for their eventual new discoveries and it's always fun.

INCUBATION

This is no more and no less than what happens when an embryo and a sperm get together and rendezvous in the womb where they incubate. The old cliché that the baby is cooking in the oven is what happens to all the information you took in during the Preparatory Phase. Everything you read, imagined, perceived, visualized and just chanced upon is now in your psychic womb waiting for the next magical phase to appear.

In general, this is a period of unknown and unlimited time where what you learned sinks into the unconscious and fuels your creativity. There is no need to become concerned about what the information you accumulated will do for you. Just let it percolate until that special moment arrives when all will be revealed. Don't dwell on your ideas hoping a solution or revelation will take place. It is much more likely that such an event will happen when least expected.

And when it happens you are literally transported into the third phase.

ILLUMINATION

The moment of the "ah ha" or "my golly", or "unbelievable", or "where did it come from", "didn't know I had it in me," or "it's about time." Finally, the inspiration or dream or the flash of insight or revelation strikes you. Whatever you call it, your discovery or creation has arrived. A new invention, theory, painting, poem or the ideas for a book or article pops into your mind. That flash of insight gives you new self-knowledge and a deeper understanding of yourself. You might call it an epiphany, spiritual awakening or revelation. This is Illumination.

VERIFICATION

The baby is born. The idea has been converted to an actual product. Usually the creator is alone when she has put the final word in her book or the final stroke of paint to her painting or the final concept in her new scientific theory. She basks in her glory and heaves a deep sigh of relief that it is finished. She can see the results of her creativity.

This is also the time when your invention, book, poem or painting achieves external recognition. 'How beautiful, what a wonderful poem, what a great idea.' This final phase gives "proof" of the value of your creation and validates its presence.

Remember that the birth of your idea is the successful ending of your search. But although verification must primarily satisfy you, depending on what your product is, it must also include the acceptance of others. Thus there is always the possibility that your creation is not appreciated by others. Every creator accepts the possibility that even the "best" idea may fail.

If a product does not measure up to expectations, the creator goes on, hopefully without any strong negative reactions.   Disappointment   is   understandable,   but afterwards the realization that one has the capacity to be creative should produce pleasure and an inner impetus to go forward.

I can't leave this subject without also mentioning that many, if not most, creations are for the creator alone and for a small group of people around him. As a result, the external recognition or lack of it is unimportant. The creative act alone is so satisfying and rewarding that external accolades are often inconsequential.   Becoming a creative person in as many ways as possible will be so stimulating that it alone will be conducive to making your senior years unique and alive.

Methods - Techniques to Make You Creative

What can you do to become more creative? Maintaining a very positive attitude toward your development as a creative person is at the top of the list. Having a number of techniques and methods to foster this development comes in a close second. I'd like to introduce you to a number of specific techniques and methods that I believe will nurture your creative spirit and broaden your understanding of the creative process. I have used these exercises successfully with many patients and in teaching creativity to small groups.

The exercises to develop creativity are manifold.   Be active. Be decisive. Be imaginative. Believe in your ability. Never stop because of doubt or the belief that what you produced is not up to par.   Remember that most creative people go over and over their works as they modify and revise them. Writers edit and reedit. Composers spend much of their time revising and improving their works. Even Beethoven spent a great deal of time editing and changing his compositions. From his notebooks we learn that he continued to rewrite the last movement of his ninth symphony until it had reached the form recognizable today. Even one of the most extraordinary creators of all time didn't always get it right the first time!

Before starting the exercises I suggest that you read or reread the addendum at the back of the book on the

Introduction to Mental Imagery. The use of mental imagery is one of the best ways to influence your mind. It has been used for centuries and we know today that it actually causes physiological brain changes commensurate with those formed in actual physical activity. I also suggest that you use a journal, either the one that you may have already started or preferably a new one to keep a record of your imagery exercises, as well as other activities that you pursue as you expand your life. We'll start by examining the obstacles that may stand in your way.

What Blocks Creativity

1. Believing that your work is useless, bad, juvenile or just not worth the effort to improve it.
2. Fear of failure. Believing you lack the capacity to be creative. A part of self-doubt that can interfere with all your positive endeavors.
3. Procrastination. Often due to one of the above but often a behavioral pattern that is present in many of one's activities. Doubts are often manifested by procrastination.
4. Filling your day with too many activities that can stall creative efforts that require time for fulfillment.
5. Giving into emotional reactions, such as, sleepiness, anxiety, feeling down or blue (depressed), restlessness and others, which occur whenever you consider pursuing a creative interest.
6. Inner self-criticism based on attitudes of parents, teachers and peers.
7. Imagining that all your productions will be judged.
8. Measuring and comparing your ability to others, which can lead to self-doubt.

Overcoming Blocks in Creativity

If you have blocks in any of your creative pursuits here are a few suggestions and techniques to immediately break them.

If you are sitting before your computer and trying to write a story or staring at a canvas unable to start your painting or gazing at the flower beds in your garden instead of planting a few flowers, you have creative blocks. I am going to repeat what I had said previously as the simplest way to overcome the block. Do it as soon as you realize you have a block. No waiting until you hate yourself or berate yourself for stalling.

Go for a Walk

Go for a brisk five minute walk. Imagine your head is clear, that you're feeling buoyant; have no, emphasis on **no**, guilt or negative feeling about your ability to be creative. Near the end of this period focus on feeling very positive and say to yourself that you will now return and start to write or paint or engage in whatever activity you were doing.

If, on returning, the same block reappears, repeat the above. You can do this three times, for a total of fifteen minutes. At that point change your entire daily schedule and do not repeat the desired creative effort. Rather start something entirely different. At the end of a given time, perhaps an hour you can return to your creative interest and try again. Many blocks are removed by the simple method of changing your behavior and thinking.

Mental Affirmations

Another solution is to set up a series of mental affirmations that you repeat frequently all day. Such an affirmation would go something like this. "Whenever I sit down to write I will immediately be able to write with abandon and without stopping. Ideas will flow and my writing will proceed easily and meaningfully." Repeat this simple affirmation many times each day.

MENTAL IMAGERY

A third solution is using Mental Imagery.

EXERCISE NO. 14: OVERCOMING WRITER'S BLOCK

Go into a deep state of deep relaxation.

The imagery setting: Imagine sitting before your computer with your hands frozen, tied or paralyzed. (Symbolic visual expressions of writer's block). Feel yourself unable to write a word.

Suddenly there is a spontaneous flash of light and your block is lifted. Your hands become lose, free of any restriction and with great speed you type away and ideas spill out of your mind. You then say, "Whenever I sit down to type I will never again experience writer's block."

EXERCISE NO. 15: CONFRONTING YOUR CREATIVE BLOCK

Some people decide they want to force the issue by actively confronting their creative block almost as though it were another person. They scold, berate or even vilify it for causing misery and torture.

Imagine you are facing a resistant, unyielding and determined person who resembles you, but is outwardly obstinate and defiant. This 'you' has decided to not be creative. You are facing a wall of stony silence. You stare strongly at this blocked part of yourself and shout defiantly at it, "You are no longer part of me. You will not stop me from being creative and fulfilled. You are out of my life!"

Exult in your power to overcome your negative self, knowing you no longer have a creative block. Don't hesitate to reinforce the imagery with a positive affirmation such as, "I will never be creatively blocked again."

One patient using this approach conjured up over a period of several weeks a literal barrage of verbal attacks on the blocked part of himself. His imagination was quite amazing. He would shout, scream is a better word, at his blocked self, calling it a "terrible totally unacceptable invader of his mind." Or he reached into himself and grabbed this bad self and immediately attacked and destroyed it.

At times he turned this undesirable self into mythological creatures, some resembling gargoyles or dragons. The animal would leap from him and they would fight long and hard until he won. He told me the exultation he felt as he valiantly struggled and eventually destroyed the animal. After each attack on his blocked self he felt better and relieved when he was able to overcome it. Within a few weeks he must have berated his blocked self twenty or more times a day, and using this technique alone, he was able to overcome it. Once you believe that you are the conqueror, almost any technique will work. Actually, when you fully believe in your ability to overcome your blocks you won't have any, which is why you need a method to get free of this barrier to your creativity.

EXERCISE NO. 16: WRITING FROM YOUR VISUAL IMAGES

Here is a very simple method to overcome inhibitions and blocks in creativity. Sometimes it is all you need, especially for writers. As you sit before your blank monitor close your eyes and spontaneously see an image appear. Describe it in detail and as it unfolds just type out whatever you see in the image. No one can keep their mind blank for long; an image will always appear. It may not be what you intend to write but it will start the writing process.

Do this each time you sit at the computer when nothing seems to happen. Slowly narrow down the subjects to those that interest you. After a period of time you will produce your intended subject and be able to write your story.

Be consistent with whatever way you decide to overcome blocks. Believe in your ability to do it. Accept that there is no such thing as a mental block in anything that you do. There are always solutions to overcome all mental obstacles. One patient, Susan, told me that what worked for her was deciding that whenever she had a block in writing her book she would take a ten minute exercise break.

She felt that the benefit from the exercise gave her a positive feeling and, even as her body was improving with the exercise, so was her mind and mental power. As Susan's physical strength increased, her mental blocks lessened. Finally, when she was exercising up to an hour and a half each day, based strictly on feeling mentally blocked, she was able to break the back of her mental block. She believed that she had converted her physical power to mental power. And just as she could do more push-ups and crunches she could now exercise power over her unruly mind, which now came under her control.

By the time Susan conquered her mental blocks she had established a strong motivation for physical exercise and continued to maintain her physical prowess by setting up a new and vigorous exercise program, a valuable side benefit from her efforts.

Types of Mental Blocks

Mental blocks come in many forms. You don't have to sit in front of a computer unable to type. You may want to write but never find the time. You find excuse after excuse to avoid writing. Procrastination becomes your second name. Excuses range from shopping, taking care of the kids, meeting friends, talking on the telephone, watching TV soaps, reading too much, constantly redecorating the house, lingering over meals and being lost in thought. None of these activities are bad. It's just that most of them could be reduced, eliminated or controlled freeing up time to write.

If you just can't seem to eliminate any of your time consuming activities this may be evidence of a mental block that isn't immediately obvious. If you believe that may be the case here is an Imagery exercise that might help you.

EXERCISE NO. 17: IMAGERY TO STOP WASTING TIME

If watching too much television or reading too much or just being lazy seems to be taking time from your wish to write, try this Imagery. Imagine that you are sitting watching TV when the television set explodes casting debris all over you and a hideous monster comes out of the debris and pounces on you. You are scared beyond belief. Even if you don't feel scared, pretend. Act the role. You want to influence your mind to make television less palatable.

Suddenly you awaken to the fully accepted realization that you can overcome this monstrous beast and with a great show of strength you grasp it in your powerful hands and throw it from you or you break its neck and kill it. Exclaim in a loud and committed voice that you will never watch TV excessively again. It will never stop you from being a highly creative person. Exult in your newfound power and know you will become a highly creative person.

If you prefer a less negative Imagery exercise, imagine that you are watching the TV and find that you can't concentrate. You become sleepy and can't fully awaken. You feel that the TV controls you. You then raise your arm, point to the TV and command that it goes off. You get up, feeling powerful and happy that you have broken the tie to the TV. Your affirmation might be simply, "I'll never excessively watch soaps or television again."

Always keep in mind that when you use Imagery, you put strong feelings into it and you believe in the power of your mind to transform you. Be persistent! No matter how many days or weeks you practice the Imagery, be patient and you will find a change in your behavior. If you encounter resistance to doing the Imagery remember that you are doing them to change thinking and behavior. Your mind knows the intent and it works because you want it to work. The exercise depends on your mindset, your belief in the process and the concept.

The techniques to overcome procrastination are similar to methods described above. Here's an effective Imagery exercise for those who tend to procrastinate in various activities, not only in developing creativity.

EXERCISE NO. 18: OVERCOMING PROCRASTINATION

> Imagine that you see yourself as lazy, incapable of getting started and you feel very guilty or angry at yourself. Suddenly, someone gives you a swift kick in the pants or lassoes you and pulls you forward or pushes you from behind. You laugh at yourself and feel buoyant and in control now that you are moving forward. You say strongly, "I'll never be lazy or procrastinate again."

Using Imagery is conducive to stopping whatever behavior is holding you back. Not only are you changing your mental state and brain but your self-esteem rises. Creating an image of what you want to do will promote positive thinking and behavior. It's a win-win approach to improving mental health and creativity. Imagery may seem silly, like a game. But it's a serious and effective technique and it can be fun.

To develop the belief in your creative self and enhance the creative spirit I'd like to present you with a series of simple but effective Imagery exercises strictly for developing your inner creative resources.

EXERCISE NO. 19: INNER GROWTH—SWALLOW A SEED

> Imagine swallowing a seed and visualize it settling in your stomach. A variation can have someone, like a God come and place the seed on your tongue. You swallow it. As you watch, you see it take root in your stomach where it

quickly grows larger and larger until it has become a small tree. It continues to grow and the branches extend from your body and head and grow larger and larger. You feel the exuberance and know that you are witnessing the awakening of your creative spirit.

You are the writer, producer and director of your images. If you don't like your spontaneous imagery, change it! There is one caveat in doing so. Try to understand what you don't like. Is there a resistance to facing some issue? Perhaps it's too colorless or it is unclear. It can be productive to stay with the imagery and try to develop it. At another time you can use the same setting and go through the imagery again. It is almost always different the second and subsequent times.

EXERCISE NO. 20: CHANGING BODY PARTS

You imagine watching your body while fervently wishing to become a highly creative being. As you stare you see different body parts change. Your arms become wings. Then they change to the front legs of a horse. Your legs become the back legs of the horse and you see yourself galloping through a meadow. You see another change as your body becomes a fish and you glide effortlessly through water. You know that you have the capacity to change yourself in whatever way you want. Your mind has developed the power to create body changes.

EXERCISE NO. 21: CHANGING YOUR IMAGE

See yourself in rapid sequence change into all sorts of animals or strange figures. See yourself as you are and then watch your face change into different characters. Hear yourself speak with different voices and different feelings.

You can use these ideas whenever you're looking for new ideas to write or paint. You can transform yourself and/or any part of your environment or even the stories you read. Your creativity will unfold as you experience the excitement and new freedom.

EXERCISE NO. 22: CHANGING YOUR AGE

Imagine yourself as an infant or small child growing into adolescence and adulthood. As you undergo these Imagery exercises you will become more spontaneous and free.

Now imagine seeing your mother and father in front of you and engaging in conversation with you as you change your age and size. You can also imagine their changing to become what you desire. As you see yourself change as you interact with them, carefully watch all the faces and bodily movements. They will often reveal attitudes and behavior that will surprise you. You can actually overcome many residual problems between you through these exercises.

Your conscious imagination controls imagery although it draws from the unconscious mind. This can help you understand the meaning of your imagery. The unconscious mind becomes a great tool for insight and can lead to changes in your thinking and behavior. Insight is the door which you must open in order to understand yourself. It becomes a tool for self-analysis. Letting go and being very spontaneous when you create this imagery will be especially helpful toward gaining insight.

Trust in your creative unconscious. It won't let you down. You will always get meaningful images, even when you use the same imagery setting. Each attempt at creating Imagery will be different as you can change day by day, if not minute by minute. Imagery follows your mood and where you are mentally.

Creativity is so important to life that no effort is

too much in developing it. It is a force of integration, helping you to overcome perceived deficiencies and becoming mentally more agile, outspoken, and less afraid.

Creativity and its Relation to the Birth Process

Creating art has long been considered a symbolic version of giving birth. Being unable to create is akin to sterility. Just as women frequently go to any length to have a child, artists will also go through much soul searching to find ways to achieve symbolic birth as evidence of their creativity. Not giving birth to a child (art) is likened to being dead inside. Producing progeny (art) is evidence of aliveness and immortality.

Many people who feel creatively blocked and are unable to find direction frequently become strongly pessimistic. Their inner struggle is projected onto the world, which they view as hopelessly floundering, or, worse, caught in an unsolvable quandary. Sometimes they fight to help to improve the world conditions that especially disturb them. In a sense they have displaced their efforts from overcoming their own blocks to joining others struggling to change the world.

In an extreme case someone who feels the world is coming to an end is often struggling with a belief that his inner self is dead and thus his world has come to an end. His battle to become creative has led to a dead end. We have an unfulfilled and unrealized person. Our purpose in this book and especially in this chapter is to assist people to overcome all negativity and become alive with enjoyment and purpose as a creative being.

The following Mental Imagery exercises can help you in your efforts.

EXERCISE No. 23: BREAKING OUT OF YOUR MENTAL PRISON

If you are feeling stymied, imprisoned and unfulfilled you are living in a mental prison and need to get free.

Imagine yourself in a tiny cell. There are no windows or doors. You are imprisoned. There are many ways to become free. Here are a few.

You are determined to get out and with sheer strength you punch a hole in one of the walls and walk out. You are free.

You take a very deep breath and exhale with such force that that walls of your prison expand and you stand free.

Through sheer mental power an intense laser beam shines forth from your mind and burns a hole in the wall. You walk to freedom.

End with an affirmation that you freed yourself from your blocks and inhibitions and will never allow yourself to be imprisoned again. You are a fully realized creative person. You did it through the power of your mind.

Each of these exercises gives you super strength to break through any walls that surround you. You believe in the power of your mind to free you from your stagnant state.

EXERCISE NO. 24: FREEDOM FROM PARALYSIS

You're in a barren and isolated place. You are paralyzed and can't move any limbs. You desperately want to be free.
  Solutions:
    Out of your head springs another you, a wise and powerful you. The new you says you can increase the power of your mind by intensifying your wish to move. You can overcome any obstacles. You will yourself to move. Make it happen. MOVE! And you move and are free.

Another version is that by the power of thought you rise up though still paralyzed and put one foot before you, then the other. You continue to rapidly gain strength and within seconds you are bounding over a meadow.

You are completely free.
End with a powerful affirmation.

EXERCISE NO. 25: ENCASED IN ICE

You are in a dark room encased in a block of ice unable to move. Through your inner power you cause your body to become hot and melt the ice. Or you will the block of ice to slide outside where the sun focuses on melting it. Or you will your body to expand until it cracks the ice into tiny pieces. You revel in becoming completely free.

Again end with an affirmation.

These examples show you some ways you can symbolize blocks and give you symbolic imagery to overcome them. You only need one that you like. Use powerful emotions and exaggerate the restriction. Never doubt your ability to get free. Your mental efforts definitely influence the inner boundaries that constrict you.

Mental imagery can bring you many solutions. I suggest that instead of using only my examples you imagine your own, something that fits your feelings and condition. Believe in the power of the imagery to change your mind. Imagery may feel like magic, but it is simply a positive and effective tool to change your thinking and behavior and it works. Don't dismiss it because of its simplicity.

EXERCISE NO. 26: FIGHTING THE RESTRICTIVE PART OF THE SELF

Imagine another you, the negative or constricted you that springs from your head. You are now face to face with part of yourself that you need to fight and defeat. You are determined to win and extricate yourself from the tyranny of this part self. You are highly confident that you can win the battle and ask the other you to choose the weapons. They can be anything, even words. You see yourself in fierce combat and exult when you win the battle. Your negative self is vanquished. You see the defeated you running away or on the ground dead or disabled. It no longer has any control over you. You have overcome your negative self.

Your affirmation can be, "I'll never feel negative or doubt my ability to be strong and creative. Nothing will impede me."

All these solutions are similar. The mind always knows your intent, which in this case is to get free of any imprisonment you feel. Once you are free, your affirmation might be, "Through my own power I have become totally free of my inhibitions, restrictions, doubts and obsessions. I am a free and creative person."

The very act of using imagery sets in motion the changes you desire. By frequent and persistent use of the Imagery exercises your thinking begins to change. Imagery is a powerful tool available whenever you need it. It is filled with symbolic magic to give you the power you need. Believe in it. After all, it is your own power.

The Group Process to Foster Creativity

Many people prefer to work in groups or with a partner when they do creative work. In general, do whatever works for you. Activities such as writing usually require being alone, though some writing, like making up jokes, is often stimulated by group interaction. Screen plays are often shared by several writers. Construction art, installation art, large scale works frequently require a group of people, although the original work, often a small version of the work that will eventually be built is usually done by one artist.

Fostering creativity through group interaction is different from your natural inclinations as a creative person. What I'd now like to describe is how to enhance creativity in participatory activities. The freedom and pleasure that one can achieve this way often leads to greater individual creative ability.

Form a group. Generally four to eight people work best. There are a number of exercises you can try.

EXERCISE NO. 27: WRITE A STORY

One of the group members starts by writing the first sentence of a story. It sets the mood and locale of the story. The next group member writes the succeeding sentence while maintaining the theme and mood of the previous writer. This continues until each person has written one sentence. By mutual decision the group can end the story after each participant has added one sentence or more if desired. The last person ends the story. The story needs to be viewed as a complete piece with the intent to have a finished story. Although each person is writing very spontaneously, it is not random. Rather he is trying to develop continuity in the story line. He is relying on his empathic ability as well as interpretation of the words.

Generally the mood should be very explicit. **If it involves anger**, then it should be very clear anger. "Get out of here and never come back." Or "Come one step closer and I'll break you in half." **If it's love**, be explicit. "I would give my life for you." A word limit is imposed. Usually ten to twenty words suffices. If after a predetermined time, perhaps 15 seconds, the writer is unable to come up with a new sentence the paper is passed on to the next in line.

Nothing is said out loud until the end when one person will read the story. In general most people are surprised by the contributions of the others.

Several Variations of Exercise 27

Follow the same scenario as in Exercise No. 27, except each person writes on a separate paper what he or she believes will be the conclusion based on what had been previously written. This is a stimulating exercise as it forces your imagination to envision the ending and will also demonstrate how much empathy was at play in the various contributions.

Another approach requires that each person only reacts to the previous sentence and not to the entire story that has already been written. Thus there is greater effort to follow the initial theme since you'd like to end with a coherent story.

The same exercise can be done writing a poem or drawing a picture.

EXERCISE NO. 28: DRAW A PICTURE

Each person will take 10 to 20 seconds to add his efforts to a drawing. It can be a simple line or a complex series of lines or subjects. To foster the group creativity each person tries to visualize the entire picture that comes from the drawing being produced, generally following the lead of the first "artist." This develops empathy and intuition and fosters the individual's own creativity. If it seems like telepathy enjoy your psychic ability.

The Creation of Drama: Acting and Role-playing

Drama and plays can be great vehicles to develop your creativity. Here are a few ways to enjoy creative dramatic communication and help develop your imagination.

A great actor is considered highly creative. This is

revealed as he interprets the words of another creative person, the writer. Perhaps we can't rise to the heights of our esteemed actors but we can enjoy and learn from reading a play or script. Whether doing it alone or with others, reading out loud from Shakespeare or Chekhov or Arthur Miller can be fun and highly educational.

Try to act free and spontaneous. Go over the same lines repeatedly, using different voices and speech rhythms. You will be amazed at the changes in your voice and delivery. Put feelings into the words. Move your body, wave your arms and animate your words. Exaggerate. Don't worry about how it will appear to others. Do this for yourself. Such mental gymnastics are also good for mind and brain development. Much as a writer searches for new words to describe a scene so does an actor search for new emotions to present the character in a new and more effective manner.

EXERCISE NO. 29: CREATING A DRAMA

Group interactions can encourage many creative opportunities that will also be fun. One such activity can be developing a composite play or drama. It can begin with imagining a theme from which characters evolve or the characters can be picked independent of a theme. Let's start with the latter approach.

Role-playing

The group decides on the various characters or each participant can arbitrarily select his own character without having any idea of the content of the play. Each member of the group will take one role. For example, the group might consist of a housewife, lawyer, grandmother, teenager, teacher and an airline pilot. When there is no theme the first speaker will start and establish the theme and mood with his words and emotions.

Keep in mind the theme can be anything. Our purpose is to learn how to develop spontaneous interactions to nurture your creative spirit. In this exercise everything is verbal. No writing. The length of each comment is decided by the group. Up to one minute seems like a workable time period. However, for different experiences the group can decide that it can be very short or much longer. The individuals watch a clock but try to estimate the time. If one goes overtime there will usually be some member who warns the speaker to end. Some variation in time is not crucial compared to the spontaneity and interaction. There is a 20 second allotment of time if a character does not say anything. The next character then takes over.

One of the characters starts the drama. Let's make it the teenager. He does not give any clues to what he's thinking. There are no explanations of anyone's intent or meaning. He says, "I think our football coach should make the governor do what he wants."

The housewife picks up the theme. "That governor won't listen to anyone. He'd make mincemeat out of your football coach."

Grandmother chimes in, "We'll march on the state capitol and lie down in the streets to stop traffic if he goes ahead with his plans."

Thus the play unfolds. It can go on as long as the group wants. The total time is generally decided before the play begins. Perhaps each speaker will have two to four times to speak. Four times would give the length of the play 24 minutes at maximum with six participants. Keep in mind that some of the speakers will only speak for a few seconds in their allotted one minute time period. Each character tries to maintain the developing theme yet has the freedom to say anything. Since empathic interaction is involved it should follow the mood and theme as close as possible. Since everyone hears all the comments silences should be limited to about 20 seconds. In the last round a conclusion must be reached.

What do you gain from this type of experience? You learn about character transformation, a new way to achieve a creative outlet. You work toward completely identifying with your character. Act, talk and be that character and say what your character would under the circumstances of the unfolding drama.   It will help you understand this temporary new you. In role-playing you can change your voice and appearance. You can give the temporary character a new life very different from yourself. It's as though you come alive in another body and mind. There is no right or wrong. You have become another person and you thrive and rejoice in your characterization.

If you want to write a novel, then you need to fully identify with all your characters and make each one alive. Every writer is a composite of the characters he writes. He reflects the lives of every character in the book. If you're a man and you are writing about a grandmother or a baby or an infant, be that character. Creativity is nourished by a conscious awareness of role playing, much as it happens with professional actors.

A group creating a spontaneous drama can pick a theme and decide all the characters will fit that theme. Say it's a romantic comedy and the six members of the group decide that they will represent three different romantic couples who meet in a restaurant. One couple can be teenagers and unmarried but having wild sex. The second might be middle aged and discover that their young daughter, one of the teenagers, is having sex. The third couple can be grandparents and having their own lively affair.

Different scenarios can evolve. The older man could be cheating on his partner and having sex with the female partner of the middle-aged couple. Or the older couple decides to split up or get married. Makes no difference. The idea is to spontaneously develop the theme. Pour yourself into the material. You'll be very surprised at the acting ability that many of you have. You can become other people without planning or even thinking how you're doing it. Your creative unconscious has taken over. This experience can be much fun and turn you on to another component of your personality.

Another variation of identifying with the different characters is taking over each other's roles and creating a new play based on the same theme but with different actors playing the roles. Each member can become all the other characters. Then as the same theme is played out you will discover totally different scenes and reactions and moods. Each person has brought his or her own personality and ideas into the life of the character.

Some older people discover a great interest in acting and join acting groups or even start one with older friends. People can then meet periodically and act out real plays. Shakespeare, Neal Simon, Chekhov, O'Neill and Arthur Miller are good authors to consider.

Other seniors discover a hidden ability to act and create plays and may take up screen writing or play writing. Besides being a lot of fun, these experiences can actually provide a new venue for many seniors.

If you review the stages in creativity you can see how this type of interaction provides the ingredients for the various phases-**preparation, incubation, illumination and verification**. As each person speaks, the others are absorbing and taking in the ideas, moods and meaning of what the other characters are portraying. These components of the interaction are continuing to incubate. When it is time again for you to speak there is spontaneous illumination and you speak freely and uninhibited. The next speaker verifies that you have brought meaning to the group. Your creation was accepted and acted on.

Two-Character Plays

Another variation is that two members of the group play a two-character play and the others watch and critique the play. They'll observe the participants' freedom, genuineness, dialogue flow and individual expression of mood and theme. One person sets the theme and mood.

"Say lady, move over. You're taking up too much room on that bench."

"Is that anyway to speak to a lady?"

"Just move over. I come here everyday and you're sitting in my spot."

"Well, that's too bad. Find another seat."

"Get up, before I throw you off. You dumb broad."

"Just try and touch me you SOB and I'll be the last person you ever touch."

You can see how the theme and mood continues and depending on how long the dialogue is, it can become increasingly violent or suddenly take a conciliatory or loving tone. Whatever comes, the other follows suit.

Acting in Pantomime

Individuals in a large group can have very creative experiences acting out moods and themes in pantomime. Initially acting without words may appear daunting but after lots of laughs from fumbles over roles you will quickly improve your techniques. This is wonderful fun and you can do it without even thinking how it might be useful in developing your creative side.

When you are home alone, stand before a mirror and become another person. Make faces to create moods, change body posture, gesticulate, exaggerate and trade in your gender and age, all without words. Every mood, every characterization, can be mimed. You'll get a kick out of this process and will recognize that you are feeling unusually creative in your efforts. Then you'll feel more prepared when you appear before the group.

Pantomime offers another dimension to personal creativity. You tune in to internal feelings and become more sensitive to your body and to your mind's awareness of your body. Since most creative efforts are mind and body related it is easy to see this as a useful technique to do alone. Empathy is improved and intuition becomes more sensitive. These experiences also intensify one's creative spirit and enliven a sense of self.

Two People Groups

All the ideas and directions for larger groups suit two people groups as well. Since many people live as couples it gives you a wonderful opportunity to find new and very special meaning in your relationship. You are already a group and well attuned to each other. Now you can expand the way you interact. Because you're always together you can do it frequently and for short periods. Imagine doing a play a night before dinner or before bedtime. These plays can increase intimacy and sexuality. Nothing prevents you from making such plays a part of foreplay even before you hop into bed.

When only two people comprise the group, roles can be reversed, or new roles more quickly adopted and the theme of a play modified or changed. The rapport you normally feel can induce a deeper and more spontaneous interaction. The time of each session can vary giving you flexibility, which is less likely in a larger group.

Couples and Theatrical Works

Couples can also play out the various characters in established plays. Each person takes over several of the roles. Keep in mind that part of this experience is changing voice and facial expressions as you play the different characters. Some couples decide to go through the works of Shakespeare alone. Some take turns picking out favorite plays and soon discover another area of interest as they pursue dramas to act out.

Many couples who begin this way go on to develop groups comprised of close friends that allow expanded play acting. Very often this occurs without any conscious thought to developing one's own creativity. Of course that happens anyway. What the couples feel are increased aliveness, a new and important activity and added spirit to their lives.

These experiences are all winners in your basket of activities. You now have the time and the wish to make this the most exciting time of your life. These are some of the ways to do it.

EXERCISE NO. 30: OVERCOMING CREATIVE BLOCKS BY ROLE-PLAYING

> If you are sitting before your computer unable to think of something to write imagine you are another person and write what that person will say. If you want to create a certain mood do it much as you did in the pantomime role. Just as it worked in the exercises for learning to role play it can work under other circumstances.

EXERCISE NO. 31: ASSUMING THE IDENTITY OF A MASTER ARTIST

This exercise requires that you know with some degree of intimacy the lives of certain artists that you admire and have viewed their works. Learning about their lives and ideas will be essential in "borrowing" their creative identity.

> To foster your creative development as a painter you imagine being that artist. You act out and mime being him before you start to paint. You strongly imagine being that person. Incorporate everything you know about the artist into your personality. Then you actually stand before your canvas and paint as though you were.

Don't worry that your work won't look like Rembrandt or Hockney. You're not trying to be them or create like them. You're trying to become more creative and are using the role playing technique to facilitate your development. By identifying with a highly skilled artist you are taking into yourself your awareness of his exceptional talent. Through repeated affirmations that you will retain his great skill, you cultivate the belief in its happening. "Whenever I become El Greco, I will absorb his wonderful talent and paint with greater skill." Much as you took over roles in plays or in spontaneous role playing, you are now taking over the role of a real person.

The same technique can be used in any of the arts. How about creating a song or poem? You can identify with a songwriter or a poet. Does your newfound creative urge stimulate you to write a novel? Countless novelists await your absorbing their writing skills and creative bent.

Occasionally someone asks me if this won't lead to plagiarism when you write like another writer. The answer is NO. Writers and artists frequently copy styles as a learning tool. It is easy to distinguish your own signature style from others. Plagiarism is deliberately taking the words of another writer and using them as your own. Creativity is the opposite. You believe in your own ability and bring forth what is your own unique self.

By now you certainly recognize that there are many methods for overcoming obstacles and stimulating the development of your creative self. Use what seems best and always be willing to experiment with other techniques and ideas, especially if one is no longer working. Your imagination and desire to increase your creativity are your primary tools to give you what you want. There is no limit to what you can conjure up with your mind. Here are a few more ideas that you might want to consider.

EXERCISE No. 32: EXPANDING YOUR MIND THROUGH FANTASIES

> Do the following mental exercises while in a state of relaxation. Sit quietly and allow your mind to spontaneously develop these fantasies. You can do them sequentially or linger on just one or two. Each fantasy can last seconds or many minutes. Visualize them as clearly as possible.

- Imagine building a house, room by room.
- Decorate the house.
- Look at a blank wall and paint a picture on it in one minute.
- Come to a barrier in the road and with a

mighty leap, jump over it and see yourself in an entirely new land.

- Swim underwater and discover incredible caves and beautiful fish.
- Become tiny and enter your body by either being swallowed, going into a blood vessel, or by being inhaled.
- Create other selves that will speak to you with new and often unknown voices. You can engage in dialogues on any subject. You will be surprised at what you know.
- Paint a picture, walk into it and follow wherever it takes you.
- Become a bird and fly into the sky. You can even fly to another planet or universe.
- Meet various animals on the road or in a forest or even in your home. Talk to them. Ask them questions, lots of questions.
- In one minute create an entire play, all the characters, the theme and the conclusion.
- Create a more complex play. Take as much time as you want. But do it all in your mind.

REFLECTIONS

You can create unlimited imagery that will not only facilitate your mind's growth, but will also give you new insights. You will discover that by doing many of these imagery exercises new ideas will readily appear and many will become material for actual artistic productions. Many stories and paintings are started with visualization and only when the artist is satisfied is it put on paper. The visual mind becomes a testing venue as well as a creative one.

Never struggle with creating imagery. If one doesn't work try another. If no images come into your mind stop and go for a walk or do something else. You should never do anything that causes barriers or hesitation or procrastination. You can always change your thoughts and behavior to facilitate your becoming freer.

If possible, always examine why a particular thought or

idea caused a block or obstacle. After all, your objectives are to get freer, more creative, more inwardly fulfilled and have fun. You have already learned that blocks are simply minor barriers that can quickly be eradicated. The day will come when you no longer have blocks, since any hesitation is immediately followed by the use of one of your many techniques to overcome them.

With the knowledge that you are now free and unfettered, you will never again be burdened by blocks. You will always have something exciting to do and will feel your creative self expanding. This is the mindset and belief that you now carry with you.

If anything contrary appears you have the knowledge of multiple techniques to change or eliminate it. You are floating on a cloud of your imagination and the world has opened its wonders and secrets to you. You can never be bored or lack interests or awaken in the morning wondering what you will do. Instead you will be filled with so many ideas and interests that you will spring from your bed with the alacrity of a child—eyes shining, singing a just-made-up song and pinching yourself. If you don't feel the pain of the pinch then you haven't really awakened, so start over. After all, isn't that the prerogative of the creative soul? Unlimited and inexhaustible and growing younger by the minute. You have discovered the mental elixir of life, the proverbial fountain of youth and you did it all with your creative imagination.

Chapter Ten

EXPLORING YOUR INNER SELF

Everyone has inside of him a piece of good news. The good news is that you don't know how great you can be! How much you can love! What you can accomplish! And what your potential is!

—Anne Frank

It is not by muscle, speed, or physical dexterity that great things are achieved, but by reflection, force of character, and judgment; in these qualities old age is usually not only not poorer, but it is even richer.

—Cicero

Your senior years can be a time for self-exploration, a time to become aware of your hidden and forgotten self. Childhood dreams, old interests, lost skills, buried talents and a deeper connection to your inner self await you. New experiences often lie just below the surface of your conscious mind. You only need to access them. Within us lie the sources of both the creative imagination and the obstacles and conflicts that burden us.

Since most of this book examines ways to establish positive attitudes and engage in pleasurable activities, it is important to focus on removing any obstacles that might interfere with our realizing those goals.

Inner Fears and Conflicts

Within your hidden self, inner fears and conflicts may exist. They may limit creativity, inhibit freedom, diminish openness to love and curtail adventurousness. Except for conscious fears that occur when we sense an immediate threat or have an anxiety state, such as facing a menacing dog or phobia, we are not always aware that they exist. At times, such inner fears can be pervasive and even dominate one's personality and behavior. Symptoms, such as anxiety or depression, without an obvious cause, indicate their presence. It is important that these issues are reduced or eradicated, if possible.

For example, a man who is consciously unhappy and despairing, who deliberately avoids people, works at home in front of a computer, watches TV alone, and has no real friends may fit this category. Without a significant person in his life, it would seem, he is living a very restricted and lonely life, yet feels incapable of changing his existence. His lifestyle may be related to unresolved conflicts from his past. His unhappiness is the clue that inner fears may be dominating his life.

A lifestyle of aloneness does not necessarily indicate underlying conflicts. If a person has no negative feelings about a life of solitude and is symptom-free we could assume that the adaptation into a life of solitude was successful.

As you read the following case history of Sharon and Warren take note how easily they made a radical change in their relationship and lives by honest and open confrontation and dialogue.

Sharon, age 64, holding tightly to the arm of her 36 year-old son, Warren, entered my office. She immediately asserted, "I am very upset about my son's refusal to leave home and live by himself. He feels miserable. Don't believe him when he claims he is happy and doesn't need to see a psychiatrist."

Sharon turned and looked at Warren's placid face. "And you need to know how hard it was to get him to come with me today." she said emphatically.

"What compelled your mother to insist that you see me?" I asked Warren.

"She feels that I'm wasting my life being alone and not seeking friends or a wife," he responded.

"And you don't see that as a problem?" I queried.

"Not at all. I decided a number of years ago that I want to live a life of peace, piety and solitude. I'm happy with my life and spend my days working at home, in order to make a living. I spend much of my time meditating. Do you find anything wrong with that?"

I looked at him carefully and cautiously replied. "No, not at all, if you're happy
Are you truly happy?"

"Yes. Very happy."

"Then why did you follow your mother's insistence to come here?"

"Doctor, you have to understand I'm a peaceful man and would not want to hurt my mother. I assumed that you would validate my lifestyle since I'm at peace. I hoped that my mother would then leave me alone."

"Warren, you know that's not true," his mother retorted. "You never go out, never meet anyone and you absolutely refuse to find an apartment for yourself. You certainly make enough money to do so."

I again looked at Warren sitting in front of me serene and at ease. I detected no obvious conflicts. On the other hand, Sharon seemed ill-at-ease and agitated.

"Did you come to see me only because your mother insisted?" I asked him directly.

Warren replied without any hesitation and no change in his mood. "I came because my mother is driving me crazy. All day long she harangues me, interrupts and criticizes me. I sometimes think that she's trying to drive me from our home, but I like it there. I have a private section of the house with a separate entrance and since I like to live alone there is absolutely no need of my moving."

I turned to his mother. "If Warren is happy with his life why did you come here?"

"Because he's lying. How could anyone be happy the way he lives?"

"Mother, if anyone is unhappy it's you," Warren blurted out. "I love the way I live but you never seem to know what to do for yourself. I've often thought that's why you bug me. Actually you've never insisted that I move out. As a matter of fact I always felt you wanted me there. I'm about the only friend you have."

A new wrinkle in the situation, I thought. "Is that a consideration?" I asked Sharon.

For a moment I thought I saw tears in her eyes. "No, not really. I stay at home because Warren is always there and he may need me."

"Mother, I am very self-sufficient and don't need you around the house. Despite your belief I do have several friends that I see. Why don't you tell the doctor why you seem so sad all the time?"

I looked more intently at Sharon. She seemed to shrink into her chair. There was no doubt that she was struggling. "It's because I suffer for you," she said in a barely audible voice.

Warren looked at me and shook his head disbelievingly.

"Warren," I said, "If you're comfortable speaking freely with your mother here please tell me about your background and current life."

"Mom, is it OK if I'm totally open?"

"Yes, of course, tell him everything," she whispered.

Warren spoke unhesitatingly. He informed me that during his childhood his mother was domineering and highly critical. She expected only the highest grades and would not tolerate any resistance or rebellion. He learned to deal with her by always giving in to her control. For years he harbored anger and took it out in sports and picking on smaller children.

His mother looked down but otherwise showed no reaction to his words.

Eventually in adolescence Warren began to go to retreats and learned to meditate and accept a passive and non-aggressive lifestyle. He attended college and studied literature and computer science. Over a period of years he became well known for his computer skills and easily found work that he could do at home. He continued his meditation and spent time at retreats and with other spiritually minded people.

Slowly he withdrew from all external activities and remained at home working at his computer, meditating, feeling increasingly spiritual and at one with God. As I discovered, he maintained some contact with several monks and a few former friends. It became clear that he withdrew from society by choice.

"It took me years to achieve this inner state of peace and contentment," he said. "But even today when my mother interrupts me I still feel a slight resurgence of anger. She's always expressing something critical about my life or wanting me to meet someone or do something against my wishes. She wants me to be different," he said softly.

He momentarily paused as he reflected on his next words. "I believe I'm able to tolerate her trying to change me since I've put up a wall to shut her out of my life."

"That's what you do to me," Sharon said to me. "Shut me out."

"Mother, I don't want to do it, but you make me. You won't leave me alone. You stay around the house, doing nothing. At least I'm always busy. I'm a peaceful man and want to live a peaceful life. Mother, you're the one who is unhappy. You cry at the drop of a hat. Sometimes you just stay in bed all day."

"I can't help it,"

By now I realized that Sharon had unwittingly come here because she was the one who needed help. She lived in denial of her real life.

"Sharon, do you want to tell me more about your own unhappiness?" I asked cautiously.

"Doctor, it's about Warren. If only he'd meet a nice woman and get married and have children, I'd feel fine."

I'm sure that would help," I said encouragingly. "Anyway, why not tell me about your life and what besides Warren makes you so unhappy."

She remained silent.

How long have you been single?" I asked.

"About twenty years," she whispered. "My husband had

a sudden heart attack and just died."

Have you had any other relationship with a man?"

"No, I needed to take care of Warren."

"Are you lonely?" I asked gently.

"Yes," she murmured, as tears now streamed down her face.

Without further questions Sharon poured out her life of emptiness, loneliness, fears of rejection, even fearing to see doctors who might pronounce her incurably ill. Her fear of losing her son's love and guilt knowing that she was so disruptive in his life had become the dominant themes of her impoverished life. Her dependent relationship with her son had become the barrier to finding an independent and more fulfilling life.

"Sharon, would you like to find more peace and happiness in your life?"

"Yes," she said softly. "Very much."

"What can you do to make it happen?" I asked.

"I can leave Warren alone and try to make a life for myself." So she knew, I thought. Change should come easy for her.

"I've always been lonely," she continued. "Even when I was married I was so dependent on my husband that not having him around was almost like being dead. I've been so thankful that Warren stayed with me, although I was really upset that he also was alone."

"I have always understood that Mom needed me to fill her life. I guess that did play a part in staying with her, although now I just find it convenient. I save money and if I ever wanted to bring someone here I could do it without her even knowing."

"I never considered that Warren was happy being alone since I was so unhappy," his mother said. "We never talked about it before."

"Can you now?" I ventured.

For the remaining time in this first session and, as it turned out, their only meeting with me, Warren and Sharon spoke freely about their frustrating existence with each other. They had never enjoyed conversations, going out to dinner or to a movie or taking a trip together. Dependency, neediness, guilt, fears of loss and rejection and especially the emptiness and lack of love in their lives had controlled their existence.

For many years a warm, intimate and even fun-loving mother-adult son relationship had eluded them. Change was about to happen. By being direct, open and friendly, Warren and his mother quickly resolved to never revert to their old ways. Sharon decided to pursue a new life and quickly saw the potential of going out to make new friends, joining some charities, engaging in some art project and even joining a gym. She assured me, even as they were leaving, that what she had learned would become the impetus for her new life.

Five or six months later, Warren wrote to inform me that his relationship with his mother had markedly improved and she was remaking her life. Instead of being controlled by her anger and depression she began taking steps to lead a more fulfilling life in her senior years. Warren's mother made new friends, including several men, and sought new activities, attended senior citizen activities and began to study painting.

Warren added new friends and activities to his life. He joined a group of Buddhist monks and acolytes to share his meditation and thoughts. Within his increasingly satisfying spiritual life Warren had expanded his world. He began to discuss his philosophy with his mother and discovered the pleasures of taking her out to dinner, something he had not done for years. With his mother's support he decided to continue to live in her house, although moving out was being considered.

From the story of Sharon and Warren two factors become clear. Intimate relationships can hide major conflicts that exist in each individual. Personal freedom depends on resolving those conflicts. Once resolved, individuals can seek and find new and highly rewarding venues and activities. Warren had made a decision to lead a life of solitude but the underlying conflict with his mother limited his true happiness. Sharon's fear of an independent life coincided with her son's wish to live a relative life of solitude.

Most importantly, and this is essential
in all age groups, never ignore conflicts

that you struggle with no matter how much you believe they do not interfere with your lifestyle. Only you can know what needs to be done and only you can fix it. The first rule to finding a fulfilling and satisfying life in your senior years is to always face all conflicts and do everything you can to overcome them. Your rewards will be many.

Stopping Negative Behavior

Many people live and die without making any attempt to cast aside the boundaries that have inhibited their behavior. They have curtailed their activities much of their lives. They might have been afraid of public speaking or lived with a social phobia while functioning behind a façade of reaching out to people. Frequently this is facilitated by medication or alcohol.

Some believe they can no longer learn anything new and even fear forgetting what they know. They no longer trust their memories or even their judgment. They have begun to withdraw into a cocoon. For them life is narrowing instead of expanding. Such inhibitions and negative behaviors need to be stopped in order to prevent developing a diminishing life instead of an expanding one.

Psychotherapy may be helpful for those seriously impaired by fears, anxiety, social phobias, compulsions and inhibitions. If you need professional help, don't short-change yourself by avoiding therapy. It can be beneficial. However, I don't believe it is necessary for most seniors. Instead with a little effort and a change in thinking and behavior you can learn ways to improve your life.

There's no point in carrying fears any longer. You're now in the second half of your life and you want it to be as fulfilling as possible. You need to decide that the emotional baggage you have carried is no longer welcome.

Here are a few suggestions that anyone can use to become freer and more self-directed. You have to carefully assess your attitudes, thoughts and behavior. Unless you are clear about what's bothering you and what you would like to change little can be accomplished.

Often, what we believe comes from the external world is really from us. For example, if you live in fear that getting in a car and driving will get you killed and therefore you no longer drive, you need to carefully assess the cause of the fear. If you were in a car accident and seriously injured, the trauma could make you afraid of driving. If the fear has no real basis, however, then it is caused by some inner belief that has been displaced onto driving. The fear of driving is then a symptom of some inner conflict.

A similar reasoning is behind most people's fear of flying. Such fears are frequently tied to the fear of dying, or a fear of being in closed spaces or losing control over your life. At times the fear of heights can lie behind a flying phobia.

Flying Phobia

For example, a patient, Caroline, came to see me for treatment of a flying phobia. In the past she had controlled her anxiety related to air travel through the use of tranquilizers but lately they had proved ineffective. Rather than try stronger drugs she was sent to me. The technique to overcome phobias can be done through desensitization which I'll explain later.

About five years earlier Caroline had been accosted and thrown to the ground. She screamed and fortunately the man fled. However, she became afraid of going outside without someone accompanying her. She needed to feel protected. As a result of this fear she started to run for exercise believing she could outrun someone if accosted again. The need to feel in control of her life intensified. Whenever she lacked this control such as driving in traffic, especially on freeways, she became anxious. She needed to be able to stop the car and get out if needed. She realized this was foolish and overcame that fear through sheer willpower, but seemingly out of nowhere her fear of flying began. Symbolically flying had come to mean that she no longer had control of her life.

Although traumatic events can lead to various phobias,

many, if not most of them occur without any discernible conscious cause. Whether you know the cause or not, a simple desensitization technique can frequently help a person overcome the condition (see below).

Some phobias are more difficult to overcome and a period of psychotherapy might be helpful.

If your fear is not related to an accident, then conclude that it comes from within and is connected with something from your past. By accepting that the fear is inwardly derived you may begin to have ideas and even clear insight about its cause. Also trust your willpower to overcome anxiety even if it has been a lifelong burden. Even a slight reduction in your apprehension can markedly improve your life. By believing that your fears can be changed, you can facilitate eliminating them. Most important is taking an active position in attempting to eradicate any undue anxiety or symptom.

Overcoming Phobias

If you have a flying phobia, you would write down all the elements that frighten you. We sometimes call this a hierarchy of symptoms. The following are potential situations that could be part of your flying phobia. Calling for reservation, leaving your home to go to the airport, getting in your car, arriving at the airport, getting on the plane, taking off, flying and landing. Any or all of these situations could contribute to a person's flying phobia. Whatever it is, imagine that particular scenario and as soon as you feel anxiety totally relax your mind and body using whatever method you prefer. This approach works for most phobias.

I have found that the **rag doll technique** works well here since it's easy to do and fast. Many people just **take a single breath** and will themselves to relax. Whatever technique you use, maintain the relaxation until you no longer feel anxious. Repeat that particular anxiety situation until you no longer have anxiety. Then go to the next situation. Continue until you have reduced or eliminated anxiety in all the components related to your flying phobia. This approach may take several or more weeks until you are free of anxiety. It works and has been used for years under the name of **Systematic Desensitization**.

The following exercise is useful for this kind of situation and for all types of fears. It differs from many of the other imagery exercises since it requires repeating the same imagery of your fear and reducing it by relaxation (Rag Doll). Once a specific fear is eliminated you do the same desensitization with other fears.

As with a flying phobia other phobias may have a hierarchy of situations that contribute to the anxiety. Consider anxiety about approaching strangers, going into crowds, public speaking or being in closed spaces. Break your fear into its components and try the desensitization process.

EXERCISE NO. 33: IMAGE AWAY YOUR FEARS

> Visualize what frightens you. When you feel the related anxiety, immediately take a deep breath or use the Rag Doll technique and imagine yourself totally relaxed. Use images of a safe and comfortable place far away from your fears. Continue to breathe quietly in the absence of anxiety. After ten to twenty seconds of anxiety-free relaxation repeat the exercise.
>
> Again visualize the object of your fear and initiate the relaxation response. You are essentially connecting the phobic situation with relaxation, which often reduces or overcomes the phobic reaction. Try doing it ten or more times a day. This exercise may help you reduce any fears and tension that impede your life. Continue the exercise until you have attained relief.

The same technique can be used for other phobias, such as fear of insects, snakes, cars and animals. Some phobias such as fear of open spaces or appearing in crowds or in social situations may be more difficult to overcome and require longer and more persistent efforts, but you can certainly reduce the fears, if not eliminate them, by persistent use of the method.

Like many of the techniques I've described in this book the essential ingredients for making changes are motivation, persistence, believing in the approach and believing in the power of your mind. Keep in mind that these exercises have been used for many years and are helpful, but they don't replace medical or psychological treatment, if needed. Always evaluate your needs carefully and take whatever steps are necessary to overcome any problems that exist in your life.

Depression

Feeling blue, excessively sad or even moderately depressed? As seniors we face accelerating losses in many areas, in addition to the loss of a job. In general, a period of mourning and grieving occurs when loved ones are lost, money problems arise or we develop a serious illness or suffer an injury. Time is necessary to assimilate the pain from such losses. Eventually it is important to adjust to the loss and end the mourning. Even grieving over the lost of a loved person ultimately must end or the life of the mourner takes on a negative cast.

It is essential that guilt, emptiness or resistance to initiate change does not impact on our ability to overcome reactions to loss. Otherwise we begin to suffer from various symptoms that threaten the happiness we seek in our senior years. Various exercises to change our moods through changing thinking can help overcome depression, sadness and other disturbing feelings.

At times the loss of a spouse, child or a parent is so enormous and the grief so overwhelming that seeking professional help is advisable and helpful. You don't have to always believe that you should be able to overcome all suffering without help.

I'd like to present a series of case histories of older people and the exercises they performed to help overcome their various symptoms.

Death of a Husband

For the past year, after 43 years of marriage, Jan, a lovely 72 year-old woman, suffered from a lingering and seemingly irresolvable depression following the death of her husband, Gary. The relationship had been complicated by Gary's drinking, his staying out late and occasional unexplained absences. Nevertheless, during 45 years of marriage, they shared many things, including four children.

As her therapy progressed she quickly recognized that she was ambivalent toward Gary, alternating between love and hate for him. Her unexpressed anger had been stymied by guilt due to her frequent wishes for his death, as well as fear of his retaliation. However, on the positive side they enjoyed satisfying sex and a pleasant social life. She was conscious of all these feelings and wondered why she just couldn't get him out of her mind and get on with her life.

During the second session we developed several Mental Imagery exercises that she intended to use to help overcome her depression. I explained the nature and technique of using imagery, including the need to exaggerate what needs to be changed.

EXERCISE NO. 34: OVERCOMING DEPRESSION

Imagery setting: Jan imagines herself cloaked in black, sitting on the floor, tears streaming down her face and looking totally disheveled. She feels completely overwhelmed by her depression and can't imagine living any longer. Suddenly a brilliant blaze of light comes out of nowhere and envelops her and she is instantaneously free of her depression and now feels joyful and completely upbeat. Her depression is over and she feels ready to conquer the world. She states that she is no longer depressed and feels happier than ever in her life.

EXERCISE NO. 35: EXPRESSING ANGER

> Imagery setting: Gary comes home in the middle of the night, drunk and verbally abusive. Jan had waited up and confronts him when he enters their house. He immediately swears at her and tells her to get out of his way. Instead she stands her ground, raises her fist and yells back. She castigates him for his excessive drinking, playing around and frequent disrespect. She imagines looming above him without fear and venting her anger until he apologizes. She accepts it and asserts that she'll never allow him to belittle or put her down again. She feels exhilarated and raises her arms to the sky and bellows out that she is well and is ready to take on the world.

Jan remained in therapy for about six weeks, learning to accept that she had both positive and negative feelings toward her husband. She continued to practice the imagery exercises and added four others to improve other areas of her life that included overcoming inhibitions about public speaking. She had always wanted to study acting and felt speaking in public was necessary as a prelude to acting. She was much improved at the end of her treatment and believed that the exercises were helping her. She said she would continue them indefinitely.

Evaluating Alzheimer's Disease

Cliff, a spry 67 year-old man, was referred to help him overcome a belief that he was developing a rapid and early onset of Alzheimer's disease. He first noticed his condition about six months ago and it had progressed to its current more "advanced" stage. He had become depressed as he perceived that his memory was rapidly declining despite psychological tests and a neurological clinical evaluation that said he was normal for his age. He had become obsessed with the fear of his descent into the Alzheimer abyss, as he put it. "My memory is so bad, I know that it is the beginning of Alzheimer's, no matter what anyone has told me to the contrary."

He gave me many examples of things he forgot to do, how he continued to misplace objects and forget appointments. "No matter what tricks I use I always forget where I put my keys."

I performed a few clinical tests that clarified that his memory was fully intact, which I immediately told Cliff. Such tests are simple to perform as illustrated:

- I asked Cliff to elaborate on something I had told him ten minutes earlier to determine if he remembered the subject and our previous discussion.
- I asked him to see if my memory was intact by seeing if I could repeat five to seven digits that he would give me. I deliberately made one mistake to see if he caught it. It would immediately be apparent if he knew my error since he would have had to also recall the numbers.
- I reversed the procedure and asked him to repeat a different series of numbers that I gave him.
- I gave him a series of nouns and told him to remember them since I would ask him to recall them later.

If anxiety interfered with the testing and if further reassurance was needed that he was not becoming senile, I performed an additional test to show him the intactness of his memory.

I gave Cliff a list of commonly known numbers, such as Social Security, license plate, telephone number, driver's license, telephone number of best friend, business telephone, etc and asked him to select one so I could check his memory of the numbers backwards. That tested both his recall of the list and also his selection of a memorized number that he should know perfectly. Whatever he picked out I knew his memory had to be fairly intact, otherwise he would not have remembered the list. Also repeating a well known number backwards is normally not difficult, but it does require an intact memory. I again reassured him that my objective appraisal indicated that his memory was normal.

If the testing indicated a real possibility of mental decline there would have been a need of further testing of brain function, either performed by a neurologist or geriatric specialist.

You can use these tests to test your own fears of losing your memory. Alzheimer's disease becomes fairly common when we reach our eighties. No one knows the cure yet, but there is some evidence that keeping your mind active with mental exercises of any kind will help ward off memory loss. Also physical exercise apparently delays the onset of mental decline. This is no time to dwell on future illnesses or handicaps. We will face our future in the most upbeat manner possible and deal with all problems quickly. Above all, live with a positive and totally upbeat attitude. This is the time for fun.

At the end of my testing it was clear that Cliff was emotionally disturbed by an imagined memory problem, which is common with people as they begin to experience normal memory changes as they enter their senior period of life.

Memory loss from early Alzheimer's is different, since it quickly gets coupled to poor judgment and strange behavior that may include wandering away from the family house and having no recollection of how to return or forgetting that one lives in such a home. It is also quite common to not remember the uses or the names of various objects.

Although Cliff was relieved by my assessment he felt vulnerable to slipping back. Previous assurances also did not last long. He remained afraid that losing his memory would cause him to lose control of his life. He worried about his declining memory's impact on his day's activities, the affect on his family, especially his wife and his fear of having a shortened life span.

We arranged a brief period of psychotherapy that included setting up several imagery exercises to help overcome the fear of having Alzheimer's. Over several months we focused on psychological reasons that might contribute to his fear.

Following losing his job two years earlier, Cliff had suffered severe gambling losses unknown to his wife and he was worried about being discovered. At that time he noticed the first signs of memory loss and realized that there was no way he could gamble again. For the short term he had sufficient money to meet financial needs but his overall retirement plans had been decimated by his gambling. He became obsessed with trying his hand once again at the gambling tables in Gardena but was terrified that he might lose again.

He tried desperately to put his misfortune and poor judgment aside but guilt and fear of exposure tormented him. Gradually his memory problems intensified and he became totally preoccupied with becoming senile. In a sense his belief that he was losing his memory preempted his guilt over his gambling losses. His obsessional state prompted his family doctor to send him to me for evaluation.

The therapy focused on his underlying guilt, fear of his wife's anger, and his somewhat precarious financial situation due to his compulsive gambling. I added several Imagery exercises to facilitate his therapy. They are useful for any kind of obsession or doubt over self-control.

EXERCISE NO. 36:   OVERCOMING A GAMBLING OBSESSION

> Imagery Setting: Cliff imagines that he is sitting at a card table in Gardena and struggling to avoid putting all his remaining money on one poker hand. He is bombarded by the stupidity of such an act and feels his brain is about to explode. Overwhelming guilt and fear of losing torment him. He feels his brain is liquefying under the assault and he visualizes his deterioration into a brainless empty shell of a person.
>
> He finally places his hands around his skull, squeezes, and, in one heroic gesture,

sends rays of light into his brain, destroying his obsessions. He feels free, his brain reconstitutes and all guilt and fear are gone. He knows and states with confidence that he is free of his gambling obsession and will never gamble again.

This imagery exercise can be modified and used with any obsession.

EXERCISE NO. 37: INFERIORITY and GAMBLING

Imagery Setting: Cliff imagines that he is a coward, an empty buffoon, and fearful of admitting failure. He believes that anyone who gambles isn't worthy of love or respect and this adds to his sense of worthlessness. He visualizes himself as a tiny misshapen figure cowering and hiding behind a chair. Finally, he looks up and imagines a force pulling him up and a voice saying that he has the power to overcome all those feelings and become a worthy and lovable man who would never gamble or do anything unworthy. He stands up and grows to an enormous height as symbolic of his newfound power and sense of well-being. He states he'll never do anything that will lead to a state of worthlessness again.

EXERCISE NO. 38:   RESOLUTION OF A GAMBLING COMPULSION
(End-state Imagery)

Cliff visualizes himself walking into a classy casino past the roulette, crap tables, blackjack tables and other enticing games. He gloats as he feels no pull toward any gambling and smiles as he quickly hurries from the casino. Cliff walks down the street feeling joyful and knowing that he has total control over his life.

Headaches

CASE HISTORY

Headaches are a common symptom that many seniors suffer. Migraines, cluster headaches, tension headaches, throbbing or pressure headaches can all be modified through reduction of tension, anger, guilt and inferiority feelings. Unresolved emotions tend to give rise to various psychosomatic symptoms. Headaches are among the most frequent reactions to stress. Always consult your family doctor to make certain there is no physical cause for your headaches.

Clare, age 68, was referred for psychotherapy when all medical attempts at controlling her moderately severe tension and migraine headaches failed. Since her divorce some 20 years earlier she had suffered from depression and frequent headaches. Her depression seemed to be controlled by anti-depressive medication but her headaches continued. Although Clare said she was never really free of headaches, they did vary considerably in intensity and frequency based on activities, interactions with her children and friends and times when she was alone and isolated.

At times, her migraines could be incapacitating often necessitating isolating herself in bed where she remained until the headache abated. Sometimes an entire day would pass. During such periods she would often reflect about her background, her former marriage and why she felt afraid of people. She knew she avoided her own anger and the many people who stirred up this feeling in her. Unfortunately her insight had no positive curative influence on her headaches.

Certain statements she made indicated a powerful underlying anger that remained toward her ex-husband. "He tried to turn my two boys against me and for a long time they ignored me and seemed to only love their father. In recent years they have been much more affectionate and spend more time with me but I can't get over what he did to me."

She retained anger toward both parents, especially her father who was away a lot and often ignored her when he was home. She seemed unable to stand up for herself with powerful men, including her ex-husband. Guilt and fear of losing love were predominant factors in her inability to express negative feelings even when it was appropriate. She internalized her anger, which manifested as tension and migraine headaches. Headaches had become her punishment for the guilt she felt. "I feel terrible having all this anger toward my father. I just can't seem to forgive him. I can understand that my headaches are punishment."

After pointing out the above connections of her emotional state and the headaches I helped her set up a series of Imagery exercise to practice at home (see below). I only saw her three times during a six week period. Afterwards we arranged that she would write me monthly for half a year to let me know of her progress.

EXERCISE NO. 39: RELIEVING TENSION HEADACHES

> Clare imagined the large claws of a giant bird tearing at her scalp and head. At times it felt like the bird was going to pull the scalp off her head. With a Herculean effort she reaches up and grabs the bird by the neck and wrenches it away killing it in the process. She exults as she sees the dead bird at her feet and is now totally free of any pain. She states that she'll never have headaches again.

Variations: Although this symbolic imagery fits Clare's feelings about her tension headaches there are many other ways of visualizing headaches: a raging fire burning in the skull, a clamp being tightened around the head or someone smashing at your head with a sledge hammer. The images to fight them include a hose to put out the fire, overcoming the person tightening the clamp or tearing it off your head or overcoming the person using the hammer.

EXERCISE NO. 40: FIGHTING MIGRAINE HEADACHES

> Clare imagined a raging fire within her skull causing unbearable pain. She felt that her brain was being consumed. Suddenly with newfound power she found an enormous fire hose and sprayed water upon the fire immediately dousing it. She felt exultant knowing that her own power had conquered her migraine. She stated that she would not let anger or any other feeling cause her to have headaches again.

Other images that patients have used include a large tumor growing inside the skull (from a patient who felt that would be worst thing he could imagine), small rats eating the brain, the brain blood vessels expanding until they burst the skull and firecrackers going off repeatedly (from a patient with cluster headaches).

Migraine and tension headaches differ although they may have similar psychological components that can be modified by therapy and mental imagery. There are certain vascular changes that may cause or accompany migraine headaches, such as dilatation of the cerebral blood vessels. Although these are underlying physical changes they are influenced by the imagery exercises.

The mind influences illnesses that may even be primarily physical or organic in nature. Don't let any belief that your headache is due to physical or genetic factors persuade you to forgo the use of mental imagery. At the very least it can do no harm and may give you lasting benefit.

You should never assume that the use of mental exercises is a substitute for evaluation and proper medical treatment of any headaches or medical condition. Even if imagery only reduces the frequency and severity of your headaches, especially migraine, you would have accomplished much. Many patients continue with their medical treatment until the results of the imagery are manifested. Discuss these matters with your physician and always use good judgment in your pursuit of any new approach to your symptoms.

EXERCISE NO. 41: HEADACHES and ANGER

> Clare visualized a huge man throwing daggers at her and making her scream with pain and anger. With an arousal of incredible power she rises up and catches the daggers in her hand and deflects them back at the man striking him each time. She gloats over her power to stop his torturing her and making him writhe in agony for hurting her.
>
> She states that she'll never be affected by any person trying to hurt her in any way again.

This imagery is directed against what is perceived as the cause of the headaches. By attacking and defeating a symbolic image of the cause the headache is no longer needed.

EXERCISE NO. 42: HEADACHES and GUILT

> Clare imagines sitting in a corner pressed against the wall holding her head in her hands, crying and believing she is the most evil person in the world and deserves to be punished severely. Suddenly a voice from above softly speaks to her and says she has suffered enough. She was not at fault for all the anger directed at her and she no longer needs to blame herself for anything that occurred in her life. She rises up, cleansed of any fault and feels free and pure. She knows that she'll never need to suffer again.

Headaches have many causes and each person who decides to use imagery as a way of reducing pain should conceive imagery that fits the individual feelings and the type of headache.

As with all other imagery, you practice the exercise

when not in the midst of the headaches. Mental imagery is a mind conditioning exercise and needs to be in a quiet state of relaxation.

I learned from Clare's monthly letters that her headaches slowly disappeared. Within four months she was almost completely free of her tension headaches, although she had occasional flare-ups of her migraines, though much reduced in frequency and severity.

Clare followed the pattern of other migraine patients that I treated over a number of years. About a third stopped having them, a few had no changes and the majority had varying degrees of improvement. I encouraged all those patients to continue the imagery indefinitely.

In addition to treating her headaches, Clare created over a dozen other imagery exercises that addressed her difficulties in becoming more social, learning to be a good cook, having people over for dinner and, above all, to overcome her depression.

She had become devoted to her imagery exercises and performed them up to 20 to 30 times a day. With imagery, more is better.

The additional imagery exercises that were effective in diminishing her depressive reactions were quite simple.

- One was seeing her face with a big sad look and taking her hands (symbolic of her mind and squeezing it into a smile.
- The second was walking down the street and saying hello to various people she would meet. She actually did this one in real time and found that, when she smiled at people and said good morning, a friendly greeting was returned that made her feel welcomed and uplifted.
- The third imagery was seeing herself dressed up and being admired by others, knowing she looked good and attracted people.

Imagery, no matter how simple, is effective because of the underling desire to change. Although imagery works by changing brain patterns and mindsets, the act of thinking positively itself creates the outlook for your future. You expect the imagery to help you and that by itself is constructive to further improve your life's situation.

Clare continued to progress and a letter I received two years after her treatment had ended indicated she was free of headaches and her depression. The imagery that helped her could have been learned without psychotherapy.

She had met a number of new friends, was enjoying her painting classes, had taken up dancing and was indeed a gourmet cook. Her relationship with her children was very positive and she had formed a close relationship with her two grandchildren.

EXERCISE NO. 43: OVERCOMING INSOMNIA-FALLING ASLEEP

> If you have difficulty in falling asleep visualize
> yourself undressing, walking over to your bed,
> lying down and immediately falling asleep.

That's all there is to it. Because it is so brief I suggest that you relax and do it three or four times each imagery session and repeat it up to fifty times a day. Do not do it within two hours of bedtime and not when you are in bed. These exercises are brain conditioners and if you do them in bed and it doesn't work you might get discouraged.

As with all imagery don't wait for it to help and do not have a time limit. I've had patients with previous lifelong insomnia that required three or more months for the imagery to work. One day you will go to bed and be surprised when you quickly fall asleep. Just keep up doing the imagery exercise. Add it to the others you are doing. All the imagery exercises should be done each session but some can be repeated more frequently. It takes very little time and there is no downside. And remember, believe in what you are doing.

EXERCISE NO. 44: OVERCOMING INSOMNIA-AWAKENING IN MIDDLE OF NIGHT

If you have difficulty falling back to sleep once you awaken, visualize awakening, getting out of bed and immediately returning to bed, lying down and immediately falling asleep. If you have difficulty falling asleep and resuming sleep, do both exercises in the same session.

EXERCISE NO. 45: MAINTAINING A HEALTHY HEART

Visualize your heart as perfectly healthy and pumping blood vigorously and slowly. Visualize the blood vessels clean, without atherosclerosis. Believe in your vitality and see yourself exercising. You know that your heart is as healthy as a person half your age.

If you have had a heart attack, visualize your heart as completely healed. Some patients imagine entering their body and floating through the heart with a laser gun and cleaning out all their arteries. You are convinced that your arteries are clear of any obstruction.

Remember imagery is an adjunctive technique and does not preclude other medically needed treatment. In most areas the medical limits may be minimal. That would not be the case for someone with heart disease. Always follow your doctor's advice and his exercise parameters. Imagery does not put stress on the heart but real exercise might.

EXERCISE NO. 46: OVERCOMING FEARS OF HAVING A STROKE

Visualize your brain as pristine, shiny and pulsating with blood flowing through it. Visualize the cerebral blood vessels clear of any obstructions. There is no evidence of any disease. You state that you are not afraid of having a stroke and you know that your brain is healthy.

Remember no one knows the future and imagery is just another way of improving the odds of your remaining healthy. We can never know what any treatment does for an individual's longevity and health. Statistics are gathered through the evaluation of large groups but can never predict what happens to the individual. Do everything possible to keep your brain healthy, including physical exercise, maintaining a good diet, avoiding saturated fats and using mental games to stimulate the brain.

There are endless possibilities for mental self-healing. Our lives are replete with struggles to make our lives healthy, vital and satisfying. Our minds can be our primary asset to foster this way of life. Or they can be the major detriment to undermine our intent to live our senior years peacefully and well. You are creating the matrix for the best years of your life. Your direction will always be toward self-healing. Always.

Chapter Eleven

DIET, EXERCISE AND HEALTH

It is exercise alone that supports the spirits, and keeps the mind in vigor.

—Cicero

It is remarkable how one's wits are sharpened by physical exercise.

—Pliny the Younger

Walking is the best possible exercise.

—Thomas Jefferson

Take care of your body with steadfast fidelity. The soul must see through these eyes alone, and if they are dim, the whole world is clouded.

—Johann Wolfgang Von Goethe

Now that you are determined to live life as fully as possible and make your senior years the best ever, you need to focus on making your body healthy, youthful and energetic. Easier said than done is the frequent response I get when I venture to suggest to patients ways to improve their physical health.

Perhaps that's true, but having a healthy body is one of the primary keys to a vigorous and vital older life. There are two pivotal elements that determine this outcome. Diet and exercise. For much of their lives many people have struggled to follow reasonable and beneficial nutritional and exercise guidelines. To some the word diet is dreaded, ignored, laughed at, or parodied. Likewise, following a structured and regular exercise program is looked upon with a decided lack of enthusiasm by seniors. Yet I believe that dieting and exercise can be fun and highly rewarding. There's little to lose and much to gain by considering a program to gain the physical health that will make your older years far more pleasurable and much longer.

Diet stands alone as a primary source of frustration in our daily attempts to improve our lives and self-esteem. Countless millions of people have tried dieting with little permanent success. Many overweight people go from diet to diet, unable to even pause to evaluate what prevents them from succeeding in losing weight. Others have given up any attempt to diet.

At first, most people lose weight on any diet, but only a small percentage of them are able to maintain the weight loss. Cyclical or yo-yo dieters abound. Enormous amounts of weight are lost each year by dieters. And it goes on year after year as the same weight is repeatedly lost. Twenty pounds lost and twenty or more pounds regained. Can this tendency, which affects a high percentage of adults who are overweight, be reversed?

The simple answer is yes. Is it difficult?   For a reasonably motivated person with a strong desire to develop a healthier body and this should include all older people, the answer is no. I have outlined a simple approach to healthy dieting that will give you abundant health, require minimal effort, and is self-directed.

We live in an era of diet at any cost. Whether you have tried one or more of the varieties of high or low carbohydrate, fat or protein diets, the results tend to be the same; initial weight loss that eventually falters and, for most dieters, a regaining of the lost weight. Most diets involve controlling calories, while some are devised around specific foods or combinations of foods. Others require specially purchased food that counts the calories for you. Some are self-directed; others involve weekly checks at a clinic by a doctor, nurse or dietitian.

Do any or all of these diets work? For some dieters they do. But too often the program ceases to function and weight is quickly regained. For others the struggle to maintain the lost weight becomes exasperating until hunger and frustration cause a relapse.

There are a number of reasons why dieting is so difficult for so many. Overweight people who have been on a number of diets, especially with rapid and prolonged weight loss, tend to develop a lower metabolic rate. Our normal basal metabolic rate that regulates our use of energy remains relatively constant with constant weight. It temporarily increases with exercise and decreases with prolonged diminished food intake. This is in addition to the gradual lowering of our metabolic rate due to aging.

As we diet for lengthy periods, our metabolic rate gradually diminishes to accommodate to the decreased food intake. This accounts for why dieters who maintain the same reduction of calories ultimately reach a point where they no longer lose weight. Their reduced calorie intake has become their normal caloric requirements. This reduction in calorie needs also accounts for why many people "eat like a bird" at the end of a diet in order to avoid regaining lost weight.

Normal or customary food intake is now considered excessive by the body due to the lowered metabolic rate. It may take many months and sometimes years before a person can eat normally. Unfortunately, this delay frequently triggers frustration and unhappiness stimulating a person to overeat as a way of compensation. The predictable result is regaining the lost weight.

Many dieters use food for filling a need for warmth, love and closeness. A feeling of emptiness leads to overeating. At times, all of us eat out of an inner psychological need. We nibble or overly indulge in some favorite food. Such eating can occasionally be tolerated provided it doesn't go on for long and a person understands how to quickly lose the resulting weight gain (see below).

The need to have special foods, especially those prepared by others, also adds to the problem of weight maintenance, when a person tries to diet without external support. Dependency on weight-loss clinics and programs diminishes the need for self-direction required for permanent weight control. Unless a diet is eater friendly, fulfills desire, taste, as well as appetite, it is difficult to sustain for long. For those on diet programs, exerting increasing control over your food choices is highly beneficial for lifelong weight control.

Finally, the word diet, as connected to weight loss, is somewhat of a misnomer. Diet should really mean the food you eat daily to maintain good health. Weight loss programs are merely a part of a good diet and are developed to help people reach an ideal weight for health and longevity.

To make dieting work for permanent weight control you need confidence and unrelenting motivation. You need to take a long hard look at your body and love it regardless of age, size or wrinkles. Since it can't take care of itself you become its caretaker. For your health's sake you must be willing to do whatever it takes to keep it fit.

Dieting for health will pay such important dividends that any effort is worthwhile. Once you understand and adapt the diet program I'm now about to present, I believe that eating for health will become your dietary norm.

WATER: THE STOMACH FILLER

Water is an essential part of the program. There's nothing revelatory about my suggesting that you drink adequate amounts of water daily. Most diet programs adhere to a similar belief. However, my emphasis is on when you drink and on not substituting other liquid beverages for plain water.

To help quell your appetite at all meals, drink a glass of water just before eating and again during the meal. This amount of liquid reduces one's appetite significantly. To prove how water works to reduce appetite wait until you are hungry and, instead of taking in any food, start to drink water. Slowly, but continuously.

Most people will lose their hunger after drinking three to four glasses of water. Some larger people may require a few additional glasses. The effect lasts a relatively short time since the water is quickly absorbed and the stomach again rumbles for attention.

However, when the water is taken in with food it remains in the stomach adding bulk and quickly helps fill the stomach, which reduces the urge to eat.

A half glass of water should also be taken with any snacks eaten outside the regular meals.

THE FRIENDLY USE OF THE BATHROOM SCALE

My next suggestion goes against the tenets of most diets and diet programs. Weigh yourself on the bathroom scale at the same time in the morning. Not surprisingly, most people who use the scale for daily weight checks hate whenever they see a weight gain. They generally hide the scale in the garage or a closet and avoid using it.

This negative attitude frequently becomes a mind conditioner implying that gaining weight is a terrible thing to have happened. The negativity breeds tension, disgust, guilt and other disturbing emotions that often increase overeating. To overcome this negativity, you must invite the bathroom scale into your diet program. It becomes a friendly partner in your attempt to lose weight and a major factor in developing permanent weight control.

Although the use of the scale is for a lifetime, it also becomes an integral part of a rapid weight loss technique. Here is the reasoning: You gain one pound of true body weight whenever you eat an excess of 3500 calories of food beyond your normal metabolic needs. However, eating that quantity of food in a short period of time would likely add between three and eight pounds of weight due to the extra salt ingested with the food. The body's homeostasis mechanism quickly retains water to dilute that salt causing the larger weight increase.

It is highly unusual for anyone except for some binge eaters to eat that much extra food in a single day. However, in proportion to the extra calories ingested, whenever you eat more calories than needed, you gain weight due to the salt content of the food and the resulting retention of water necessary to dilute it in the body. For example, if you splurge one evening and eat an additional 800 calories beyond your usual daily caloric needs, it is possible to gain one to three or more pounds in one day.

If you use the scale as part of your diet program and weigh yourself daily at the same time each morning, you will quickly learn of the added weight. Instead of despair you will know that the weight gain is very temporary and can be eliminated by the following technique. You can lose that excess weight in one or, at the most, two days by merely drinking more water than normal. For each pound of weight gained you would drink 1 ½ glasses of water beyond your normal water intake.

To maintain the body homeostasis the excess water is quickly flushed out of your body by your kidneys. The kidneys excrete the added salt with the added water and you are back to your former weight. The added one-quarter pound you gained from the 800 additional calories can also be eliminated by reducing your food intake the following day or exercising longer so that even that small gain quickly disappears.

The other primary reason to use the scale for the rest of your life is to know what your weight is and thus be able to control even small increases in weight. Eating just 250 unnecessary calories each day puts on two pounds of flesh each month. That's 24 pounds a year. An increase of just 125 calories a day, not much more than a slice of bread or one good sized chocolate candy or an extra glass of orange juice will add 12 pounds a year to your weight. It creeps up on you. You need protection. The protection is your friendly scale. This is an important mindset change and you will never get upset by any reading on your scale. The scale is your friend in maintaining weight control.

THE STABILIZATION PERIOD

Another part of your new program is called the Stabilization Period. This alone will help you control your weight loss on any diet. Simply, you diet for one month and stabilize your weight for one month. By alternating diet months you avoid the gradual decrease of your metabolic rate, which will allow you to return to a normal food intake faster once you have reached your ideal weight.

In addition, during the alternate non-diet months you will slowly learn to control your weight. The average weight loss of four to eight pounds per month is far easier to control than the larger amounts after months of dieting. A reduction of 500 calories a day will cause an actual loss of four pounds a month. By the end of your diet you will have gained considerable practice in stabilizing your weight and learning how to eat normally again. By the time you reach your ideal weight you will be experienced in weight control having practiced it for months.

During the alternate months many dieters use a journal to jot down conditions, temptations and emotional reactions to occasional relapses.

KNOW YOUR CALORIES OR USE THE SCALE

Eating without gaining weight is essential for weight constancy. If the number of calories you take in each day is equivalent to your caloric needs then your weight remains stable.

Individuals vary greatly in their eating habits. The range of calories, types of food, frequency of meals, and number of snacks depend on age, taste, gender, exercise, work and individual metabolic rates. Whether you gain or lose weight does not depend on the kinds of food you eat. Instead it depends on the calorie count.

Most people do not know the number of calories they consume each day nor the amount needed to maintain a stable weight. They need a daily measuring device, namely the scale, unless they prefer to depend on the tightness of their clothes. Since the scale is infrequently used it is no wonder that weight gain tends to creep up on people. Using a scale offers you a device to maintain your body weight indefinitely.

By using the scale you don't need to know the number of calories in your food. Taking your daily weight is your accurate and unbiased informer. However, I do encourage all people to know the ingredients, the health benefits and the calories of what they eat. The information for much of this is now printed on all foods. Knowledge of calorie input allows you to more easily regulate your diet.

A POSITIVE MENTAL ATTITUDE AND A HEALTHY DIET

Maintaining permanent weight control is dependent on two other elements. The most important is your mental attitude. First, you must believe in your ability to direct your life. Having a positive mental attitude or mindset, and a sense of optimism about your life will benefit you in many ways. Controlling your diet is just one of them.

You will be able to be more productive, creative, loving and giving. You will find ways of sharing your own bounty and receiving the offerings of others. Having a positive outlook on life and believing in your ability to change will prove invaluable in your older years.

Weight control also depends on a healthy diet. Eating for health in no way interferes with the pleasure of eating. You don't eat less and you don't eat unsatisfying or unsavory foods. You can even have desserts, if desired. However, a healthy diet helps develop a healthy body free of many of the ailments that affect older people. A healthy diet is far easier to maintain than a non-healthy one. You tend to avoid highly dense, calorie packed and fat-laden foods.

A healthy diet interacts with your positive mental attitude, since you now want to maintain your health and body weight. You also tend to sleep better, exercise more, seek activities that are more gratifying and generally live a better life. Your approach to health becomes contagious.

What is a healthy diet? We live in an era of countless diets. It sometimes seems that a new one appears overnight and tempts us to try to lose weight once more. Many diets are presented by experts in the medical and physical therapy fields. Some come from individuals who developed a diet through personal experience and experimentation. A few are replays from previous diets that have made a comeback.

How does one determine what is best and what is healthy? How can such differing diets all be healthy and effective? Can a diet that proclaims eating unlimited protein and fats be as healthy as one that believes low fat and limited protein is the way to go. Is a high or low carbohydrates diet better?

The merits of these diets have been exhaustively studied and critiqued. Rather than enter that unending controversy, I believe you should follow the well documented dietary suggestions based on the careful studies of the United States Department of Agriculture (USDA) and the Department of Health and Human Services (HHS). Their dietary recommendations follow the current advice of nutrition scientists and are followed by most nutrition experts and health institutions that include the National Institute of Health, the American Diabetic Association and the American Dietetic Association.

Simply stated, the proportion of your daily calorie intake of carbohydrates should be 55%, fats: 30% or less and proteins: 15%. If you can, restrict your fats to less than 25% and use primarily polyunsaturated and monounsaturated fats.

The bulk of your diet should be directed toward eating food that is both healthy and satisfying. By following some general guidelines you will automatically be within these guidelines. This can be accomplished without giving up the desserts you may desire.

What is different is your perspective. You are going to structure your diet to include extremely healthy and stomach-filling foods. The greater the quantity of low calorie foods that you eat the easier it is to feel full without gaining weight. The stomach reacts to the weight and bulk of the food you eat. At a certain level in your stomach you will feel full.

Vegetables and fruits are the two types of food that satisfy taste, bulk and health. From the stomach's viewpoint being filled with one pound of vegetables or fruits or one pound of meat or cheese makes little difference. However, the calories in the one pound of vegetables or fruits are one tenth to one twentieth that of one pound of meat or cheese.

OTHER TIPS FOR WEIGHT CONTROL

Certain little tricks and ways of eating also favor the lessening of your food intake. Some people find that eating an apple, chewing on celery (almost no calories), or a limited number of single raisins, carrots or individual Cheerios could become another useful dietary tool.

Chewing your food very slowly until it is well masticated decreases your intake. Cutting your food into bite-sized portions can also help.

Drinking water, as previously mentioned, helps if it accompanies all food entering your mouth.

Mindfulness also lessens eating. Mindful eating is simply nothing more that giving your total attention or concentration to your eating. You merely concentrate on every bite, the way you chew and how the food feels in your mouth. Eating is slowed down. You tend to eat less. It's a kind of eating meditation.

Rather than talk, read, watch TV or listen to music when you eat, your complete focus is on the act of eating. Some dieters use this at the beginning of each mouthful of food and after careful mastication then read or talk.

Those who want to lose weight and permanently control their weight should simultaneously use all the techniques they can think of and learn new ones. Use whatever you can to put the balance of power in yourself.

Due to the temptation to overeat sweet foods, desserts are frequently indicted as the devil's food. Although there is some truth in that assessment, desserts don't have to be eliminated from your diet. It's more a matter of selection and quantity control. Eating a small piece of cake, pie or candy is not likely to interfere with your diet. However, it is necessary to control your impulse to eat large quantities or more than a single piece.

Some dieters prefer not to eat any desserts believing that it's easier to eliminate the temptation by never buying or ordering desserts. For others, selecting less fattening desserts, such as nonfat ice cream and certain nonfat cakes and pastries presents the better of two worlds. You can enjoy delicious desserts while maintaining diet control. As you slowly move toward eating for health you will tend to find more flexibility without the fear of gaining weight.

Planning a healthy diet can be gratifying and fun when you know that you have an almost unlimited variety of foods to choose from. You'll find you can include many of your favorite dishes. The only caveat is to try and keep it within established guidelines mentioned above. In developing a lifelong eating plan you will need to consider what is healthy, what will make your weight control more effective, and what will be enjoyable to eat.

PROTEINS

Any type of protein you enjoy fits into this category. Fish, especially fish high in omega-3 lipids, such as salmon, tuna, mackerel, and others can be eaten several times a week. Meat, which includes chicken, turkey, beef, lamb, and pork, should be lean and limited to three or four times a week. Dairy products such as milk, cheese, ice cream, and yogurt, preferably low fat and nonfat varieties, can be eaten in moderation daily. Proteins in legumes, beans, soybean products, nuts and various grains and vegetables can satisfy much of your protein needs. Above all, prepare foods you like and be moderate in your use of proteins that are laden with fat.

FATS

The types and amount of fat you eat can affect your overall health and cause obesity. Less than one third of your fat intake should be saturated fats, not always easy to accomplish, since saturated fats exist in most healthy foods in varying amounts. Milk products, meats, fish, and oils made from grains (soybeans, corn, and others) have some saturated fat. Some foods such as coconut and palm oil are primarily saturated fats. Many desserts are laden with saturated fats. Try to keep your intake of saturated fats under 20 grams per day and your Trans fats as close to zero as possible.

Monounsaturated fats are the healthiest of all fats and are found in olive oil, canola oil, most nuts, and avocados. Eat even these healthy fats sparingly in order to keep your total fat intake low.

Polyunsaturated fats are also considered relatively healthy and are found in oils, nuts, grains, and fish. Be cautious in eating any food that pushes your total fat intake over 30% of your diet calories.

CARBOHYDRATES

By comprising 55% of your caloric dietary needs, carbohydrates become the most prominent part of your food intake. Preference should be given to complex carbohydrates. Refined carbohydrates like white bread and white rice are generally high in simple sugars and are quickly broken down to glucose, the primary sugar that exists in the bloodstream. Sugar in candy, soft drinks, and desserts, which often include corn sweeteners, fructose, honey, and molasses, are likewise quickly broken down to glucose. In a healthy diet you would keep such simple sugars to an absolute minimum.

Eating more complex carbohydrates, generally seen in whole grains such as wheat, oats, corn, rye, and brown rice, as well as in most vegetables and fruits, are the basis of a healthy diet. You should bear in mind that many cereals and breads are not whole grain and may be loaded with sugar. Try to use whole grains as one of your staples. They are quite delicious and add fiber, vitamins, and minerals to your diet.

Vegetables are so varied and plentiful you should be able to find many that satisfy both your palate and your nutritional needs. In general, vegetables that are colorful are most nutritious. I like to think of certain vegetables as super foods due to the many nutritious compounds they contain, such as antioxidants that protect us from cancer and other serious illnesses. They include broccoli, spinach, tomatoes, carrots, sweet potatoes, yams, kale, peppers (especially red peppers), and dark green leafy vegetables like romaine lettuce. Other less widely used vegetables that are both healthy and tasty are Brussels sprouts, cauliflower, asparagus, garlic, onions, mustard greens, and Swiss chard.

Fruits are also high on the list of healthy foods and should be a part of your daily diet. There are also a number of super fruits based on their high level of phytochemicals, the plant chemicals that improve our level of health. In general, fruits with the deepest and brightest colors are the ones to eat. They include most berries, like strawberries, blueberries, and blackberries; also melons, especially cantaloupe, Crenshaw, honeydew, and watermelon; and oranges, mangos, plums, cherries, and papayas. Apples and bananas, though not highly colored, contain many nutrients.

As you plan your diet each day, try to include as many whole grains, fruits, and vegetables as possible. They are all high in micronutrients, including vitamins, minerals, fiber, and phytochemicals. They provide most of the antioxidants we need to neutralize the free radicals that float in our bloodstream. They also help regulate many bodily functions.

FIBER

Fiber, the indigestible part of food, comes in two forms. The insoluble form increases the rate of food moving through the intestinal tract and adds to stool bulk. The soluble form, which can be dissolved in water, binds bile acids and cholesterol and may help lower blood cholesterol. Both types are found in whole grains, fruits, vegetables, nuts, and seeds. A healthy, moderate carbohydrate diet will assure the dieter of the recommended thirty grams of fiber a day. Fiber may help protect us from a variety of conditions, such as irritable bowel syndrome, diverticulitis, and colon cancer.

VITAMINS AND MINERALS

Do you need extra vitamins and minerals if you eat a healthy diet? Deficiency diseases are now relatively rare in our society. However, over half the population uses vitamin and mineral supplements. In addition, most essential vitamins and minerals are added to a variety of foods, supplementing the amounts naturally found in them. In general, those eating a healthy diet do not need most supplements, but may benefit from taking a daily multivitamin and mineral tablet. However, this is an individual matter. Becoming acquainted with herbs and vitamins allows you to determine what supplements you need to emphasize in your strivings for good health. My advice is to read for information and use caution in taking supplements. By eating a healthy diet taking most supplements are unnecessary.

Recent dietary guidelines indicate that seniors should have at least 800 IU of Vitamin D a day. Since multivitamin tablets generally only provide 400 IU it is important for people to be in the full sun without sun screen about 15 minutes a day, at least several times a week. Only a small part of the body has to be exposed to gain the benefit.

The vitamin B complex present in grains, vegetables, and fruits has a number of essential vitamins that may be supplemented by a B complex tablet that includes B_6, B_{12}, and 400 micrograms of folic acid. These vitamins are usually supplied by multivitamin tablets. Vitamins B_6 and B_{12} regulate the blood level of homocystein, a risk factor in coronary artery disease. Beta-carotene, another important antioxidant, will most likely be supplied in a healthy diet.

As with most vitamins, minerals are also added to many foods and occur naturally in a variety of foods, especially vegetables, fruits, and whole grains. Certain minerals, such as iron, are abundant in meats, beans, fruits, and green vegetables such as broccoli. Unless you have an iron deficiency disorder there is no need to supplement your food with iron.

Calcium is an essential ingredient in bone formation. It helps to prevent osteoporosis, facilitates nerve, muscle, kidney, and cardiac functioning, and is not adequately supplied by many diets. Dairy products, certain fish such as sardines, and some leafy green vegetables supply calcium. Also, calcium is frequently added to a variety of foods, including certain cereals, orange and other fruit juices, and frozen yogurt. It has been recommended that women over the age of fifty and older men have 1,200 to 1,500 mg of calcium a day. If your diet does not supply this amount you should consider taking a daily calcium supplement.

Selenium is another important mineral in the antioxidant defense system and although it occurs in various plants and nuts the amount is not constant. Daily supplementation of 100 to 200 micrograms a day of selenium should be considered.

Becoming familiar with the vitamin and minerals in foods or the amount of calories in common servings of foods simplifies your preparation of a healthy diet. Eating large amounts of the super vegetables and fruits each day will fulfill most of your vitamin and mineral requirements. Although you should strive to eat a healthy diet, you can eat anything you want as long as your calorie intake does not exceed your daily metabolic needs.

It is useful to become acquainted with the physical size of what you eat in terms of its caloric value. You should eat a variety of foods to get the nutrients you need and the right amount of calories to maintain healthy weight. For those dieters who prefer to eat foods in measured amounts the following examples offer serving sizes that can be adapted to most other foods. By serving fruits, vegetables, and whole grains as the basis for your diet and going easy on fats, oils, and sweets you will be eating the proper number of servings. Your protein needs will be fulfilled by eating your favorite sources moderately.

The following are one-serving sizes.

Milk, yogurt, and cheese group
   1 cup of milk or yogurt
   1½ ounces of natural cheese
   2 ounces of processed cheese

Meat, poultry, fish, beans, eggs, and nuts
    2 to 3 ounces of lean meat, poultry, or fish
    ½ cup of beans
    1 egg
    2 tablespoons of peanut butter

Vegetables
    1 cup of raw leafy vegetables
    ½ cup of other vegetables, cooked or raw
    ¾ cup of vegetable juice

Fruits
    1 medium apple, banana, or orange
    ½ cup chopped, cooked, or canned fruit
    ¾ cup of fruit juice

Bread, cereal, rice, and pasta
    1 slice of bread
    1ounce of ready-to-eat cereal
    ½ cup of cooked cereal, rice, or pasta

I realize that most people do not have the interest or motivation to learn what constitutes a measured portion of food and its calorie count. It's not easy to do. Many things influence the amount of calories in foods. For example, consider the following. What is a medium sized apple or banana? An apple can be 75 or 150 calories. Is your tablespoon a true tablespoon in size? Bread comes in different sizes. Some slices are as low as 40 calories. Some are as high as 110 calories. Some rolls can be 200 or 300 calories. How many calories are in a handful of almonds or peanuts or in one almond or one peanut? And do people count almonds or peanuts one by one?

Judging the size of a portion of fish or meat isn't easy. You can be off by 100%. And can you tell how many tablespoons of sauce are in your pasta dish? If it's a fat-laden sauce you can be off by several hundred calories. Many sauces, such as Alfredo sauce, have a large amount of fat. Pure oil is 120 calories per tablespoon. Many sauces approach that caloric value. A single tablespoon of sauce in a large bowl of pasta would hardly be noticed. So how many tablespoons are in it? It is helpful to practice measuring portion size and calories in all your foods, but caution and carefulness become the watchwords when judging portion sizes.

Eating in restaurants makes it quite difficult to know what ingredients are in the food set before you. Fats can be hidden in the preparation of the vegetables, meats, or sauces. Several glasses of wine that you may not ordinarily drink during home meals and enticing desserts can add many calories. People on diets try to avoid any obviously fattening food and for brief periods of time their motivation and discipline aid this control. But, as is well known, maintaining the control tends to falter and the appeal of fat laden foods often wins out. Be alert to control this temptation.

Mental Imagery and Weight Control

For many seniors the diet program I outlined may be sufficient for weight control. However, for those who find the temptation to overeat is too strong to control with diet alone, I suggest you incorporate mental imagery exercises into your weight control program.

In the following three case histories I'll illustrate how certain patients handled their diet. The diet control techniques and description of the factors that contribute to their being overweight may benefit you. Diet and weight problems are varied and thus need different solutions. Most overweight adults have tried one or more diets without success. I encourage you to consider the diet I described and add mental imagery to fortify your control. The mental imagery exercises that I describe in these cases will augment the actual diet program.

Maintaining your weight depends on using an effective diet program, and having the mental ability to control what and how you eat. The following mental imagery exercises are designed to help you develop the belief in this ability. They are one of the keys to opening the door to full weight control. If they don't work for you, drop them, but continue the diet program until you have reached your desired weight.

To make your dieting as effective as possible reduce and eventually eliminate all negative thoughts about your weight. Whether you lose weight or not, you need to like your body and avoid self-criticism. Your acceptance of your body is crucial to becoming a happy and satisfied person.

If you decide you just want to stabilize your weight, focus   on eating a healthy diet, increasing your physical well-being and developing imagery exercises to strengthen that resolve.

Health and longevity are more important than being thin. A thin person who eats an unhealthy diet and doesn't do any exercise is short-changing his or her life. Your value as a person is not dependent on your weight. Weight control is strictly another element in gaining good health and increasing your physical ability and vitality.

CASE HISTORY NO. 1

Jackie, age 64, slowly walked into my office. She appeared sweet though sad and was moderately overweight. "Doctor, I'm not able to control my eating habits and I hate myself when I keep eating even though I know it's wrong. I don't binge or eat too much when people are around. It's when I'm alone; I just can't stop nibbling. I eat whatever is handy. No special foods, just what's there. It stops me from doing anything worthwhile when I'm home. I almost have to go out just to stop eating since it doesn't occur when I'm busy out of the home.

"I don't mind being heavy anymore. I've been like this most of my life and I've been the same weight for years. I've tried to lose weight but it never works more than a few months and I put it all back on. I just have to stop all this eating. It's driving me crazy." She looked toward the floor as she finished.

"Jackie," I began, "Are you certain that you're not interested in losing weight but just controlling your compulsive eating?"

"Well, not exactly. But I've tried so many diets that I feel I'm just born to be fat. But always eating when I'm home makes my life miserable. I try to only eat things that won't put on much weight, like Cheerios, berries, raisins, one at a time." She paused and smiled knowing that must sound funny to me.

"I eat lots of fruit and cut them up into small pieces to make them last longer. Sometimes I can't help it and then I really indulge myself, especially with cookies and candy. When I'm so full I can't eat anymore I finally stop. But when I finish I'm so mad that I stop eating for a few days to lose that extra weight. I guess I punish myself for gorging. But it's all part of this crazy need to always eat when I'm at home. You can't imagine the time I spend doing this. I'm sometimes afraid of returning home. But if I didn't stay away, I'd be as big as a horse."

"By controlling your weight in that fashion it does show that you have some ability to control your food intake," I said. "Perhaps we can expand that into giving you total control over your eating. First, I'd like to describe a simple diet program that may be useful to help you control your eating. Whether you want to use it to try to lose weight again is up to you. It has several features that are different from most diets." I proceeded to explain to her the diet program (See above).

"Since you have been heavy much of your life, I'd like to introduce you to some very effective Mental Imagery exercises used by many of my patients to help them gain control of their eating compulsions. If needed, we can then look further into why you overeat since it is often related to certain emotional problems. The imagery helps you overcome the specific ways that you overeat." I described the imagery method (see addendum).

"There are many different forms of compulsive eating," I continued. "So far you've told me that you primarily overeat only at home and it's mainly nibbling although you occasionally splurge or binge. What do you feel contributes the most to your eating compulsion?"

Jackie thought for a few moments and said, "It's not the kind of food since I'll eat whatever is available. The impulse is with me all the time. I only have to go to the refrigerator and get something to eat and I'm nibbling. I do that a hundred times a day."

"So you frequently go to the refrigerator to get your food."

"Yes, or I get food from one of my food cupboards."

"Good places to start," I said, "beginning with your use of the refrigerator."

EXERCISE NO. 47: CONTROLLING COMPULSIVE EATING: REFRIGERATOR

Imagery Setting: Based on her raiding the refrigerator for food that usually precedes her constant nibbling.

Jackie visualizes going to her refrigerator eager to get food. She feels ravenous and can't wait to eat. She opens the refrigerator door and out swarm bees (she is deathly afraid of bees). Terrified, she backs away. She then slams the door shut and wraps a heavy steel chain around the refrigerator and secures it with a heavy lock. She tells herself that she'll never go to the refrigerator again to get food to compulsively eat.

Instead of bees it could be snakes, rats, vermin, or other unacceptable and frightening animals that jump from the refrigerator. It could also be something obnoxious that is in the refrigerator with the food.

EXERCISE NO. 48: as above, except using CUPBOARD.

EXERCISE NO. 49: CONTROLLING COMPULSIVE EATING—FOOD ON DINING TABLE

Imagery Setting: based on Jackie eating whatever food is available.

She enters her house and immediately sees the dining table covered with all kinds of delicious food. She reaches for some food and she is astonished to see it move away from her hand. She tries again and it again moves away and this time grows a face that sticks out its tongue and taunts her. She laughs so hard she falls to the ground. When she rises she looks at the food and says she'll never compulsively eat from any food that is on the dining table.

Variations of this imagery are many. For example Jackie could take the initiative and grab the tablecloth and shake the food to the floor or take a hose and wash the food away. Or an ax could descend and cut off her hand as she's reaching for the food. Or the table can suddenly start rocking or flying away and the food goes into the air. The results can be grotesque, horrifying or humorous.

Some patients make up imagery where the food becomes like a pet and multiplies until it fills the room and almost suffocates them. Another imagines the food letting out a terrible odor or watching fungus that grows on the food and spreads to cover everything on the table. This can be obnoxious or even humorous.

Use your imagination. You're trying to change your mindset about eating. You already know through many attempts at losing weight and trying to control your eating that it's not easy. Like all imagery you need to practice this daily for many weeks or months, and completely believe in the process and in the power of your mind to change your thinking and behavior. Never give up because it doesn't appear to be working. The imagery is just one part of your overall program and together they will work. Believe it.

Occasionally patients wonder if negative imagery will diminish their pleasure in eating. The answer is NO. The mind always knows the difference between normal healthy eating and compulsive eating. Many people who are of normal weight snack throughout the day but are able to stop whenever they desire and control the amount they eat, so they never gain weight.

After developing the imagery Jackie continued therapy and realized that her overeating was a repetitive playback of a childhood pattern. As a child her mother insisted that all the children eat everything on their plate or they would be sent to bed without the usual kiss and being tucked in. As a child and adolescent she also found it difficult to sit down at home and read a good book. Instead she ate and watched various TV programs to wile away the time.

Jackie had no encouragement from her parents. Rivalry with her older sister who was extremely intelligent and constantly put her down made her doubt her intelligence and contributed to her feeling of futility to pursue anything of value.

She had always wanted to attend college but an early marriage prevented it. I encouraged her to resume her education and attend college or some extension courses at the local high school or college. I pointed out that resuming her education is one sure way to feel younger. She laughed in anticipation of sitting down with young students.

Jackie also tried some other techniques to control her eating. Since going outside was a reliable way to stop the compulsive eating I suggested using it as a technique. Whenever she felt the urge to eat to immediately get up and leave the house. She would return after a few minutes. If she wanted to eat again she would again leave the house for only a few minutes. The object was not to stay away from the house all day but to add this to her other techniques. She would be desensitizing herself to her nibbling compulsion. If a few attempts in briefly leaving her house didn't help then she could follow her former method of staying away for the day.

She would patiently use all the techniques and anticipate the gradual reduction of the compulsion until she could remain at home all day without compulsively eating. She would not put a time limit on how long she would follow her complete program. **Time limits add a negative mindset to making behavioral changes.** It implies that you don't fully believe in what you are doing.

CASE HISTORY NO. 2

Walter, age 77, was sent to me by his internist to help him lose weight. He had suffered a heart attack and it was imperative that he lose at least 75 pounds (he weighted 290 pounds). In the past he had been unable to find any diet that would work for him. He would lose 10 to 30 pounds and then quickly gain the weight back. Now the need to lose weight was urgent and he needed a method that would give him a better chance to keep the weight off. After introducing him to the diet program we developed the following imagery based on his eating tendencies.

EXERCISE NO. 50:   COMPULSIVE EATING—BLOCKING ENTRANCE TO FOOD MARKET

> **Imagery Setting**: Based on his tendency to go to the food market whenever he wanted to binge. He kept little food in the house as a control technique to reduce his periods of binging. His normal diet between binges was actually healthy and kept separate from the binging food, which comprised large amounts of carbohydrates, TV dinners, sweets, beer and candy.
>
> **Imagery**: Walter visualized approaching the food market when he was ravenously hungry and desperately wanting to buy food. He found a huge guard holding a club the size of a tree and several vicious looking dogs standing in front of the door. Whenever he would approach the dogs would snarl and leap toward him, only held in check by the guard. The guard shouted, 'Keep away from here. This market is only for good people who eat normally. Not for you. Keep away.'
> Walter realized that the market was now closed to him and he swore that he would never again attempt to go to a market to buy food for binging.

Variations of this imagery: There can be a wall around the opening to the market. Or a wide chasm opens in front of him as he approaches the market or a wall of fire with tongues of flames leaping at him.

EXERCISE NO. 51 :   BLOCKING BUYING FOOD AT MARKETS FOR BINGING

> **Imagery setting**: In addition to presenting obstacles to entering the market, Walter also created barriers to buying food when he had entered the market. In the market he discovers that anything he wants to buy is missing or flies away or disappears when he reaches for it or laughs at him or crumbles to dust the moment he touches it.
>
> Sometimes a box will laugh at him or cajole him to laugh at the futility or foolishness of trying to buy food for binging. At the end of this imagery Walter would strongly acknowledge that he'll never go to the food market to buy food for binging.

As Walter continued to use this imagery during a period of many weeks he elaborated on his interaction with food. One imagery involved his interaction with a whole chicken. He reached for the chicken which suddenly came alive and pecked at one of his fingers. Walter tried to remove his hand and the chicken flapped its wings and flew up and bit his nose. Walter tried to swat it away and it pecked at his eyes and then pulled out his hair. Walter ran terrorized through the market pursued by the chicken.

In subsequent imageries the same chicken called up reinforcements and soon other chickens, cows and hogs, fish and eventually even vegetables were chasing him through the market. His attempts to outwit them became increasingly funny. They became like movies in his head until Walter couldn't wait until he sat down for his imagery sessions, whenever he had a spare moment at home. He told me that at times when his imagery ended he just rolled on the floor laughing.

Walter quickly stopped binging and overeating but did not give up his imagery. He proceeded to imagine other long imagery exercises that involved his wish to become a painter and an interest to resume trying to meet women, especially now that he felt increasing success that he would lose weight and heal his heart.

EXERCISE NO. 52: COMPULSIVE EATING AT PARTIES

Imagery Setting: Walter loved to go to parties and gatherings and eat all the food in sight, especially the hors d'oeuvres.

Walter imagines that he is at a party and reaches out to take a morsel of food from the passing waitress. Immediately, she draws back her hand and sprays him with water from a water pistol (she could have used a pepper spray gun or a real gun or knife) and says, 'You're not to eat this food ever again.' He backs away and realizes that such overeating is now completely over and feels good about his decision to stop this behavior.

Variations: The food can taste terrible. Or when he goes to eat it he finds that it's covered with ants. Perhaps he grabs some food, which bites his lip or tongue.

During the following year I saw Walter monthly and thereafter he wrote to me for several years. He lost 90 pounds of weight in two and a half years and believed that he no longer had any compulsive need to eat. He ascribed much of his success to the use of water as described in my diet program, the stabilization period which gave him opportunities to learn to adjust to minor periods of weight loss and to his use of Mental Imagery.

He was convinced that the imagery was the mental stimulus that allowed him to believe in his ability to make the changes in his behavior. He had created over a dozen new imagery exercises and learned to paint, enjoy exercising and dance. Walter wrote me several times during the succeeding few years to inform me that his weight control had succeeded beyond his dreams.

CASE HISTORY NO. 3

Another patient binged whenever she ate in a restaurant or

felt compelled to go to food markets to buy food for binging. Humor accentuated all her imagery. In the market the food flew around her head and even taunted her by darting in and out of her mouth. Cans would jump on her head and then pile up until they reached the ceiling and quickly topple down.

In restaurants she'd have waiters pour soup over her or stumble and spill her dinner on her dress or trip and fall on her. She even played out some sexual scenes by having food at parties sneak under the table and crawl up her leg. Sometimes they went way up and tickled her. This patient gained quick control over her eating mainly because she put all her feelings into the process and fully believed that her mind was making it clear that overeating was not possible for her.

What Kind of Imagery is Best?

I've been asked if it makes any real difference on what kind of imagery is best. My answer is to always create imagery that fits your particular eating problem and one that resonates with your feelings. Whether it is humor-filled or only uses grotesque objects or magical or even spiritual images makes no difference. The most important element is believing in what you're doing and believing in your mental power to change your thinking and behavior.

EXERCISE AND HEALTH

As we get older the importance of exercise increases. Older people tend to be more sedentary, less apt to engage in a disciplined series of daily exercises and are less involved in sports. Yet our older years are the crucial period to maintain physical fitness. If there is a known elixir of life it is exercise. Not only does it prolong life but it adds vitality and youthfulness to your age.

Exercise also helps you lose weight by increasing the amount of calories expended in a given time period. The calories burned during exercise vary considerably based on the kind of exercise, the length of time you exercise, and the degree of effort used.

In general, exercise can burn from 100 to as much as 400 calories per half hour. Although exercise is a very important part of weight control, it is not an essential part of losing weight. After all, if you exercise and burn 500 calories but then eat an additional 500 calories, the exercise did nothing to contribute to weight loss. Weight control still boils down to eating no more calories than needed on a daily basis.

However, since many dieters use exercise as an adjunct to losing weight it's important to be aware that exercise also tends to increase appetite. Thus, unless extra care is taken to control food intake when exercising it may not help in a weight loss program. Exercise will help you lose weight if there's no additional food intake, but think of exercise primarily as an excellent way to live longer, maintain youthfulness and be healthier.

EXERCISE AND CALORIES

To give you an idea of some types of exercises and their range of calories burned, I've listed several activities and approximately what a 150-pound person will burn in a one hour period.

Sitting: 80 calories
Standing: 100 calories
Housework: 250 calories
Fast walking: 300 calories
Weight training: 500 calories
Jogging: 700 calories
Running: 800 calories

If your objective is to lose weight you need to establish a daily calorie limit for your diet and maintain it on exercise days. Monitoring your weight is crucial, especially if you exercise vigorously or for prolonged periods of time. Increasing your water intake during exercise days will help you avoid eating extra food. Maintaining calorie reduction is easy if you use the scale daily. The scale will reveal any miscalculation on your part about the amount of food you are eating.

Although there is a gradual breakdown of muscle tissue as we age, exercise is the antidote. With exercise there is a gradual replacement of fat with muscle, especially with weight building. In a resting state muscle tissue burns up to twice the amount of calories that fat tissue burns. Therefore, building muscle bulk through exercise eventually becomes an important part of your permanent weight control program. At the very least, exercise can keep you from losing additional muscle tissue.

Whenever you are on a diet, you want to maintain muscle tissue and burn fat, which only occurs if your total caloric intake on exercise days is less than your total metabolic needs for that day. Fat will then be burned for energy while muscle is maintained intact by the exercise.

If you have arrived at your desired weight and continue to exercise while maintaining this weight, you will gradually change your body configuration as fat is burned and muscle is created. Muscle weighs more than fat by volume and thus your body volume will diminish while your weight remains the same.

The advantages of making exercise a lifelong part of your daily activities are many. Any level of exercise improves general health. The benefit for your cardiovascular and pulmonary systems is well known. Recent studies show as little as 30 minutes of moderately paced walking three or four times a week is beneficial for your heart. There appears to be no additional cardiovascular benefit from more prolonged and more vigorous exercise. However, there are other benefits for more prolonged exercise, such as an improvement in your ability to engage in sports and more spirited and energetic sex.

Exercise also helps control Type 2 diabetes, reduces high blood pressure, diminishes the likelihood of strokes, increases the immune system's ability to fight illness, and reduces the incidence of certain cancers, tension and depression.

Exercise helps you retain the feeling of youthfulness and slows down the body's tendency to reduce the basal metabolic rate (BMR) as you age. You can determine your BMR, that is, your minimal metabolic rate for an inactive person, by typing in "basal metabolic rate" in Google. The BMR calculator will be listed.

The body continues to burn added calories after your exercise has ended. It also increases your feeling of well-being and vitality that adds to your motivation to keep your body weight constant. I encourage you to add exercise to your daily regimen if you have not already done so.

INCREASING YOUR BMR

Many people who have undertaken diets without a stabilization period have discovered at the end of their dieting that their metabolism has slowed down and they can no longer eat a reasonably normal meal. Often, they can raise their metabolic rate by a prolonged period of moderate to vigorous exercise. I strongly suggest that you discuss this program with your family doctor, if you decide to try it. Also you should begin the program slowly and gradually increase the level of exercise.

During all exercise your metabolic rate is raised to burn stored sugars (glycogen) and fat to give you the energy needed for the physical activity. There is a tendency for the metabolic rate to remain elevated for up to 15 hours after exercising, especially when the exercise is strenuous. If you want to increase your metabolic rate, I suggest that you divide your exercise into two periods a day for up to six days a week and do aerobic exercises, such as cycling, fast walking, running, or swimming. You might wish to add weight training to this routine. Prolonged repeated exercise maintains the heightened metabolic rate.

One to two hours of exercise a day for a period of several months are needed to make a permanent change in your BMR. A less arduous exercise routine over a longer period of time can accomplish the same change. Many of the dieters who followed this program for several months were able to increase their intake of food permanently.

Generally, I don't recommend starting this specific exercise routine while on a weight loss diet program since it's difficult to assess the benefits while dieting. However, if you're motivated to add this to your overall plan for weight control, then by all means do so. Many older people who increased their exercise program reported that they had more energy, felt mentally and physically more alive, and were able to eat normally without gaining weight.

CONCLUSIONS

Developing an effective diet and exercise plan will enhance your entire sense of aliveness during the second half of your life. By seeing this older period as special and the opportunity of a lifetime, as indeed it is, you can create a new you. Eating healthy and exercising faithfully are the keys to this magical period that lies ahead.

Once you've established a program of diet and exercise make it an integral part of your life. Always eat for health first and pleasure second. This will not exclude the fun of eating since healthful eating is also delicious and unlimited in its variety of food.

Exercise should be as important a part of your life as your three meals a day. Exercise is a wonderful method of living healthier and with far more vitality. Don't let any negative thoughts intrude into the scenario of the wonders of exercise. Don't see it as a burden or a chore or hard to do.

Once you accept exercise as healthy and fun you will look forward to stretching your muscles and enjoying your newfound stamina to climb hills and run marathons. Activities that had seemed difficult will become easier. Best of all you will look forward to taking long walks, strolling the beaches and hiking in deserts and mountains. Your life will open and your mind will be enlivened. Once again I reiterate that exercise is the only true elixir of life and coupled with a healthy diet will add many youthful and vital years to your future.

Chapter Twelve

FILLING THE GAPS

Anyone who stops learning is old, whether at twenty or eighty. Anyone who keeps learning stays young. The greatest thing in life is to keep your mind young

—Henry Ford

A journey of a thousand miles begins with a single step.

—Confucius

Grow old along with me.
The best is yet to be,
The last of life, for which the first was made.

—Robert Browning

After you have settled on a healthy diet and an exercise program that works for you, there are many other factors that will contribute enormously to your well-being. **Laughter heads the list**. It abounds throughout the world. There are thousands of laughter clubs to share high spirits and fun. Laughter yoga and laughter therapy are available to humor seekers. And laughter knows no age. It's a natural for older people to want humor and pleasure in their lives. What better way to fill your hours than by laughing at life, laughing at the life that you are determined to make into your own paradise.

Laughter cures ills, raises people out of gloom, spreads joy and makes you healthier. You can laugh at jokes, funny situations, comedy acts, the antics of a kitten and even at yourself.

> *Laughter comes from a sense of wonder, openness and optimism. It comes from seeing the bright side of life and having a readiness for surprise and chance. Having a sense of humor bridges chasms and breaks through barriers in relationships. People laughing together feel closer and friendlier.*

For many couples, **sharing humor** is the single most important element that sustains their intimacy. It helps them overcome arguments and makes them laugh at foibles and missteps. It removes the irritation and grudges that plague other couples. It brings light and hope where darkness sometimes resides.

With humor you reach out and engage others. It often brings out the very best in those you touch. Perhaps even more important it helps you reach in and tickle yourself. As the old song refrain goes, "Laugh a little," and your life will take on a special glow.

The potential for humor is within all of us. It's why we laugh together at funny pictures and comedies. We laugh at the same time in humorous situations in movies and stories and react to the same punch lines in jokes. When it is missing, something in you has gone awry. Sadness, dissatisfaction, depression, insecurity, feeling unloved and loneliness can play a part in curtailing your sense of humor. Negative attitudes, seeing the world as unfulfilling and finding fault with others and yourself, thwart humor. It would appear then that any efforts to overcome negativity will be well-rewarded.

Read as many funny stories and see as many comedies as possible. Often repeated laughter will help you break a cycle of boredom and loneliness. Laugh out loud. Try to share the humor with others. Since there's no downside to this prescription for health, keep it up until it works for you. Laughing can change who you are. Try it. Nothing to lose. And it's good for you.

> *Another element to keep you healthy is remaining youthful. Think young. Think like a curious child. Think outside the box. Dare to be different. Be playful, roll on the floor with your grandchildren. Belt out a song, in tune or not. Go for a skip instead of a walk. Coach a soccer game. Barbecue the hamburgers. Be spontaneous and above all be alive.*

Most people react positively to youthful older persons. They often blurt out, "You seem so young. How do you do it?" Besides the pleasures in the recognition of their youthfulness it reminds older people that the efforts made to retain youthfulness also attracts others. So how is it done?

No surprises here. Keeping your body healthy and fit and your mind alert and active are the tricks of delaying aging and staying young. No matter what your current age you should start planning now to remain young for the rest of your life. So what if you're 80 or 90.

Youthfulness is revealed in the way you think and talk. The gestures and emotions that you bring to your conversations convey to others that you're a young person. There's excitement in your voice and bearing. Your animation and liveliness is felt and seen. The reaction is "you seem so young' for your age.

Through exercise you will be more alert, more active, walk with a springier step and move your body with a greater sense of balance and ease. You'll also engage in activities that most older people avoid due to a lack of physical fitness.

Once you get over that age is determined by a calendar the sooner you will live by your wits and body alone. That is the only true measurement of age. Be and feel young and you are young.

Another desirable and exciting component of becoming older is the opportunity to reconnect with your creative self. As children we were all creative and as older adults we still retain the potential though it is often hidden. You need to express it. Since I hold that the age of retirement has as its preeminent potential the making of all seniors into creative beings I devoted the entire Chapter Eight to the subject. Creativity that brings so much fun and satisfaction to people is waiting for you.

Become more **social**. Go beyond the many good friends that come from your past that you will always retain. Find new organizations and make new friends. Be selective and try to develop a few close and meaningful relationships—those to whom you enjoy talking and revealing yourself. You're older now and do not have to hide behind false pretenses or protect your job or even protect yourself. Although I addressed this issue before, it bears repeating. Having good friends and sharing ideas and feelings are among the bounties of being older.

Many people seek others to share **intimacy**. By joining organizations and finding sources of activities where people like yourself go you will come in contact with other seekers. Then reach out. Open up. Become actively interested in those you meet. Get to know them. Your interest in them will open doors. People react to those who show interest. In turn they will want to know you. Such mutual interest is what leads to close friendships.

Meeting **new friends** depends on being in places where the likelihood increases. Attending adult education classes in subjects you like will attract similar people. As will religious groups, charities, and environmental organizations. Go where potential friends might be. You will find new friends.

Travel more. Return to formerly loved countries and cities and find new ones. Traveling enriches the soul and brings you into contact with other people. You will find friendliness and warmth returned in kind as you reach out with your own offer of friendship. You can travel for fun, education and discovery.

Consider spending a longer period of time in new locales instead of moving too quickly from town to town. You will find warmth in your neighbors, even when you speak different languages. Reach out to them. Become friendly. Eat at their local restaurants and buy at the family markets. By immersing yourself in foreign cultures you develop a new awareness of the vicissitudes of society. An additional way to enrich your life.

Solitude beckons some and threatens others. In the first half of life most people equate being alone with loneliness. But as we get older we find we are often alone. The need to understand and enjoy your aloneness and solitude is essential to your well-being. Solitude is a state of mind that offers another way of being. It is peaceful and transports you into a different frame of mind and allows you to imagine a new and unique world, a world separate from your usual existence. You can meditate and practice the art of complete mindfulness. You can truly tune into your inner world.

Cultivate your sense of solitude. Learn to meditate. Many people who are single feel that they have reached a point in life that would have been impossible if married or living with someone. They find a special pleasure in solitude and aloneness. Thoughts spring into their minds that are new and awaken ideas and dreams. They become more creative and productive. They have freedom that can only occur when alone.

Others who prefer sharing life with another person don't have to preclude enjoying the benefits of solitude. Being older gives you options to decide on your way of life. There's an art to the practice of being within yourself. Solitude is a special state of mind. Some find periods of solitude rewarding. Through meditation, seeking periods of separateness, even when living with someone, and taking time to be alone can help you discover a new and meaningful part of yourself.

At times solitude is thrust upon us. When a partner in life dies or leaves a relationship the remaining person is temporarily abandoned. Initially depressed and self-absorbed, the person may gradually adapt to living alone and ultimately may shun relationships and love. Many times the adaptation becomes permanent. The person's world has shrunk and once the depression has lifted there is often genuine satisfaction in solitude.

Some older people choose to be alone and seek solitude. They may decide to not seek new friendships but prefer the connection with nature and animals. Others find that books and art satisfy them and living alone is peaceful and welcoming after a life of conflict and difficulty. Experimentation and a desire to enrich your life is all that's required to determine if periods of time in solitude are for you.

> I suggest that you find time to be alone and learn to enjoy solitude. It will stir your imagination and creativity. It will allow you to find the self that may have been lost as you focused on work, family and friends. It is not meant to steer you into isolation or friendlessness, but to add to your riches in these special years.

The endless bounty of nature is available to people of all ages and should be especially enjoyed by every older person. Nothing offers as much diversity and beauty and even love as nature. The splendor of flowers and trees, the songs of birds, the fluttering of a hummingbird's wings and the leaves that fall gracefully from the branches of trees overhead are all well-known. But there is more, much more.

Trees have strange and intriguing shapes and twisting branches that defy gravity and turn into caricatures of animals. They will spark your imagination. Study the leaves and awaken to their diverse designs. Touch a tree and imagine it as a sentient being. A being that may be hundreds, even thousands of years old.

Flowers are unlimited in beauty and enticement. A rose rises from a tiny bud. As you watch it grow and develop, it becomes a beautiful flower that can be cut and brought into your home. Within days you can observe the rose as it fully opens into an object of indescribable beauty. Even as you stand in awe of its captivating glory it slowly fades away and drops its petals as it returns to the earth from which it sprang.

Stroll in parks, and seek gardens to admire and savor. Watch birds fly above your head. Get to know them. Listen for their songs and whistle back. The flutter of butterflies and the scurrying of insects and tiny lizards are everywhere, yet missed if you don't look. Climb the hills and mountains that surround you. It is your time to add an immeasurable treasure to your older years. They will enrich you in ways nothing else can. You have time to bring more beauty into your life. Nature is always there and is ever faithful. It will never let you down. It is one of the true rewards of living on earth. Nature will help fill your later years.

REFLECTIONS

Is there an overriding idea or concept that can guide you into a fruitful and life-affirming older period? Perhaps each of you will determine what that is for yourself; but a number of ideas stand out.

- Strive for abundant health of body and mind. Shed the image of being an old person and replace it with the image of being a perpetually young person in an older, but fit body.

- Believe in yourself. Listen to your ideas to determine how you want to live these special years. Overcome any negativity that threatens to curtail the excitement and contentment that lie ahead. If what you're doing is not what best enlivens your life at the time, change it. It bears repeating that these years can be the very best of your entire life.

- Seek ways to express your creativity. Bring forth new ideas or find ways to interact with loved ones or discover ways to make your life more vital. Do everything possible to stimulate and retain your underlying childhood curiosity and aliveness.

- Let love be the guiding emotion of these years. Love yourself. Love others. And love the bounty and beauty of our world.

- Make your retirement years the pinnacle of your life. Just imagine the wonders that await you. Reach out toward them. They can all be yours.

FINAL AFFIRMATIONS

- Believe in the power of your mind.
- Believe in your ability to change your thinking and behavior.
- Ferret out and change all negative mindsets.
- Convert all unnecessary and unacceptable ideas into positive ones.
- Humor will help you overcome most difficult moments in life.
- Education wards off boredom and feelings of inadequacy,
- No matter how dreary life has become it can be improved through your mind.
- Act on what is truly valuable and not on what is valuable primarily to please your vanity or your neighbor.
- Read and think. Stopping either is stopping your mind.
- Physical activity helps the mind as well as the body.
- Mental imagery is a skill of the mind that directly influences the brain.
- Whatever your situation in life, accept it, but never cease trying to improve it.
- Creativity is the act of revitalizing yourself. It is a renewal of your being.
- Creativity is a way of life not only a function of producing something new.
- Love is the single most important element that gives us well-being. Don't lose it. Keep it as a treasure.
- Solitude is another aspect of the complete life. It's not just having time alone. It's how you spend that

time.

- Dream and fantasize. The world awaits the dreamer. And always look to the stars.
- Give back to those who follow you. Your future will be richer.
- Never believe your calendar age. It will deceive you. You are always much younger.
- Tell those you love that you love them. Do it everyday.
- Grandparents need grandchildren to love as much as they need you to love them.
- Don't carry any negative beliefs. They weigh on your ability to fly.
- Spirituality is a form of love.
- Music is the ambrosia of the soul. Drink it everyday.
- Your health is in your hands. Keep them clean.
- Everyday awaken with a song in your heart.
- Repeat daily that you will live in the NOW. It's really the place to be.
- Sing a little everyday. Your unhappiness will flee with the spread of your sounds.
- Dance a little everyday, even if it's a two-step, as you skip down the path of life.
- Hug a tree, and whisper to a butterfly and tell a flower you love it. They will reciprocate in spades.
- Enjoy man's creations. Art is another medicine for the soul. Look at it and then do it yourself.
- Above all believe in yourself. Love yourself. Live the dream. Even if you're 101.

PERSONAL GUIDE FOR CHANGING YOUR LIFE: A TWELVE WEEK PROGRAM

There are several ways to benefit from the exercises described in this book. You can practice those that appeal to you or you can follow this twelve week program. During this time you will learn a realistic method that will lead to a revitalization of your life. Your objective is to become a highly creative, vital, happy and self-directed person.

After this period your knowledge of mental imagery will guide you as you create your own imagery. Your expanding range of exercises will closely correspond to your growing understanding of yourself.

As part of the exercises of the 12th week you will have an opportunity to take a guided imagery tour to enjoy the new power of your creative imagination.

The practice of meditation offers you a simple but highly effective method for body and mind relaxation. I believe that each person will highly benefit by developing a daily routine of meditating, independent of other exercises. It will be the first exercise to do daily as part of your twelve week program. However, meditation can be done separately from the mental imagery exercises that will comprise the bulk of this course.

Development of the Twelve Week Mind-Expanding Program.

I will introduce a series of imagery exercises each week. As you read through *Create a Happy and Exciting Retirement* select those exercises that serve your needs. You can always change imagery as your ideas change, but eventually you need to arrive at a series of exercises, whether one or ten, that you want to do daily. Using the same imagery works best.

Imagery can be modified slightly week by week or even day by day as long as the variation is not major. It is better to add another exercise to your imagery package rather than change one that still serves your needs and delete those that no longer serve you. Find a series of exercises that work for you.

There were periods in my own life when all my imagery was directed at a serious back problem. Once the problem was resolved my imagery was directed to my creative process. At other times I used a variety of imagery to foster my personal growth and to develop inner peacefulness. Imagery is unlimited, as is your mind. These techniques will transform your life.

WEEK ONE

The first four exercises in the book introduce meditation and ways to help you become more acquainted with your inner self and familiar with the use of imagery. As you reread the exercises from the book, review ancillary comments related to them.

1. **Exercise No. 4 Learning Meditation**. (15 minutes) Once daily
2. **Exercise No. 2 Knowing your inner self** (1 to 5 minutes) A trip into your inner world
3. **Exercise No. 3 Symptom Reduction**(1 to 2 minutes)
4. **Exercise No. 4. Understanding Symptoms**. (1 to2 minutes) Listening to your inner voice

5. Start a journal; answer the following questions, daily or weekly, or as frequently as desired:

- Do I feel the exercises are working? If not, explain in writing what barriers are standing in your way. The very act of exploring the obstacles starts the process of overcoming it.
- Do I sense any resistance to completing the exercises? If so, identify what it is. What can I do to break through the resistance?
- Do I have difficulty in visualizing? This tends to improve as you practice. Imagery is effective even if you sense the picture rather than see it clearly. Try closing your eyes and visualizing an elephant. Some will see it vividly in color or in black and white while others will only see a blank screen, Most will see it in varying degrees of clarity. If you only see a blank screen, still with your eyes closed, try to draw the elephant that you "don't" see. What you now recognize is that the picture is in your head and you had no trouble tracing it. Continue to use imagery even if there is no clear picture. Most people who practice imagery do find, however, that the imagery becomes clearer with time. Either way the imagery works. Don't give up.
- Do I encounter diminished motivation? What am I doing about it? What imagery can I create to counteract it?
- Do I believe wholeheartedly in what I'm doing? If not, closely explore why not. For many it's something they need to

take on faith since the evidence of its
effectiveness takes time to occur.
Believe in it, even if you have to
pretend, at first.

- Is my imagination improving? If not, sit
quietly and just visualize and "listen" to
what comes into your mind. Whatever it
is foster it by your interest and even
excitement. Your mind is very
accommodating and will produce
pictures and movies that will knock
your socks off. Keep trying; it will
happen.

- Other meaningful comments.

- Remember, that your journal is strictly
for you. No one will ever read it. Be as
honest with yourself as possible. You
are in the process of opening your mind
and the opener is in your hands. What
a wonderful challenge!

WEEK TWO

1. Continue daily use of **Exercise No. 4. Meditation**

2. Repeat **Exercise No. 1. Knowing your Inner Self**

3. Repeat **Exercise No. 2. Symptom Reduction**

4. Repeat **Exercise No. 3. Understanding Symptoms**.

5. Exercise No. 5. **The Rag Doll**.

   This is to be done at the beginning of each
   Mental Imagery set of exercises, which you
   will be developing in the coming weeks. With
   the use of the Rag Doll you will now be
   starting your Imagery exercise routine and
   begin to use the techniques that will
   transform your life.

6. **Exercise No. 6. Changing Negative Mindsets**.

   Do **five times a day** starting with the Rag Doll. Spread the exercise throughout the day. The time will be approximately 15-20 seconds each episode.

7. **Exercise No. 7. Life as a Loving Person**.

   Do **five times a day**.
   Add this to the package of exercises that now includes nos. 6 and 7 preceded by the Rag Doll. Time added 8-10 seconds. Total time is 23 to 30 seconds for exercise package.

8. Complete journal entries.

As the program evolves you will realize that some exercises are done just once a day unless you desire to do more. Others will become part of a package of exercises that are done more frequently. Eventually this package will reach your desired number and you will have options on selection.

WEEK THREE

1. Continue **Exercise No. 4. Meditation**.

   Hereafter, I won't mention meditation in your weekly program since you will have determined whether you want to make it a part of your daily lifestyle. Meditation has many benefits besides relaxation to be considered. I strongly urge you to continue it.

2. The continuation of **Exercise Nos. 1, 2 and 3** now depends on your personal inclination.

   You can always use any imagery from the past any time you want. **You can never over use**

imagery. You will also eventually create your own. You might want to develop imagery to improve your golf or tennis game. For example: You can easily imagine improving your golf swing or tennis backhand. All artistic efforts will lead to many new kinds of imagery exercises. You will be surprised at how easy it is to create your own exercises once you have made these exercises a part of your daily lifestyle.

3. **Exercise No. 11. The Inner Sanctuary**.

    Do just once as part of the daily exercise group. This is one of my favorite exercises. It allows you to establish connections with significant people from your past. But it also gives you access to famous people, dead or alive. Although the voices come from your creative self, what you hear will often astonish you. You can gain much insight and wisdom by engaging in these conversations. I suggest that you do it whenever you want. Whether that's once a week or daily, use it for gaining access to an inner resource.

Today begins the development of your **Creative Imagination.** Since imagery must be repeated to be effective I'll rely on your evaluation to determine   which exercises you wish to continue week after week. Each week I'll list those that you should consider as part of your personal program. Today we start with four exercises. **All will be directed toward the development of a positive attitude about being creative.**

4. **Exercise No. 19. Inner Growth—Swallow a Seed**.
    The essence of creativity is believing that you have an inherent ability that will come forth, evolve and help you grow into a viable creative person. The tree is the symbol of that inner

creative self. This or some similar exercise should be part of your future imagery package.

5. **Exercise No. 20**. **Changing Body Parts**.

6. **Exercise No. 21**. **Changing your Image.**

7. **Exercise No. 22**. **Changing your Age.**

8. Complete journal entries.

If creativity is high on your list of future accomplishments I would consider doing the above exercises over a long period of time. Later, I'll describe other exercises that you can add to your repertoire depending on what you wish to accomplish. Painters would have different imagery than someone interested in becoming a writer, composer or poet.

We will use the imagery exercises to develop your creative imagination and to help overcome barriers to its realization.

WEEK FOUR

1. This is the week to work toward overcoming creative blocks. Most creative people have them at times. After a period of using imagery to overcome blocks you should be completely free of them. Also keep in mind that it is useful to add to your daily routine other ways to changing attitudes. Imagery is only one tool to help you become the vital person you seek.

2. Continue **Exercise Nos. 19, 20, 21 and 22**.

3. **Exercise No. 15**. **Confronting your Creative Blocks**.

4. **Exercise No. 23**. **Breaking out of your Mental Prison**.

5. **Exercise No. 26. Fighting the Restrictive part of Yourself**.

6. This week you are now doing seven exercises. **Time involved is 65 to 80 seconds**. I now suggest that you up the frequency from five exercise periods per day to ten per day. **Total time is 11 to 13 minutes per** day. By now many of you may be doing the exercises up to 20 times a day. The total time is a mere blip in a day's activities. For what you're getting it's a bargain.

7. Complete journal entries.

WEEK FIVE

1. We're continuing our **theme of creativity**.

2. Do all 7 previous imagery exercises

3. **Exercise No. 16. Writing from Visual Images**.

   This exercise is actually the prototype for others. If you are blocked when you sit before your canvas or in your kitchen waiting to conjure up a unique meal or need to give a talk at your local Senior Citizen meeting, use the same technique. Imagine any picture or any meal or any theme for your talk. Then follow them. If they are not quite right, you have at least broken the block. Then you can move forward, no longer blocked as you work to access the desired area that you need. Added time 8-10 seconds. Total time is 73 to 90 seconds per episode.

4. **Exercise No. 32. Expanding your Mind through Fantasies.**
   Do as many of the suggested topics as you desire or add different ones that are more pertinent to your search. **Time--1 to 5**

minutes. This exercise does not have to be done daily although it's a great one to stimulate the imagination.

WEEK SIX

You are at the half way through the program to change your life. You now have to decide how many imagery exercises you will add to your exercise package. In general, I believe that **up to ten to twelve** is a good number, which takes about two minutes for each exercise group. If you do them ten times a day, a total of 20 minutes of your time is involved. I've had patients who have spent well over an hour doing imagery exercises and some athletes who do more than that.

This program is designed to provide the impetus for developing a life-long commitment to your own growth. Today, I'm going to add certain exercises for overcoming various emotional symptoms and inhibitions preventing you from becoming a more vital person. I will add four of them. Either do a total of 12 exercises or begin to eliminate those you feel are less important. Sometimes you can combine in one exercise what was evolving in several. Play around with this.

Trust your understanding to make the right choices. After all, you can always change your mind. Just realize that you need to continue the imagery for an indefinite time. One day you will realize that you have changed your thinking in many areas and are indeed a different person. It will happen.

1. Continue the eight previous exercises or begin to make changes as described above.

2. **Exercise No. 33. Image away your Fears**.

    Time –about 30 seconds based on the need to transform anxiety into relaxation. Consider this exercise separate from your usual imagery group since desensitization takes more time. Review page 247 *Desensitization.* If it fits into your personal needs, add it to several of your daily episodes.

3. **Exercise No. 45. Relieving Tension Headaches.**

   Time—8 to 10 seconds.
   This imagery exercise can be used for any kind of headache. The imagery in the illustration was developed by a patient. Read the Variations under the exercise. You can also use a similar approach to reduce or eliminate any symptom. Your **creative imagination** will guide you to create appropriate imagery exercises for whatever symptoms you might have.

4. **Exercise No. 51. Maintaining a Healthy Heart**

   Time—8 to 10 seconds.
   Many people fear having a heart attack. Visualizing your heart as completely healthy and believing that you are influencing your body's ability to combat disease reduces anxiety.

   This exercise illustrates how to visualize your body free of any disease. Patients have also used similar imagery to overcome the side effects of medication and radiation. Imagery is to be considered an adjunct to medical treatment in helping your body heal. Does it really work?

   There is some evidence that it helps people with terminal cancer live longer and helps the immune system combat disease. Cancer patients use very aggressive approaches, such as, visualizing enormous white cells gobbling up cancer cells to destroy the cancer. Patients trying to stimulate the immune system visualize hormones (in symbolic form) and large number of white cells to fight disease. There is nothing to lose by using imagery since it's being added to other treatment modalities. For a few minutes a day you are assisting your body's defenses and immune system to work for you. Believe in it. You have nothing to lose.

5. **Exercise No.18**. Overcoming Procrastination.

Time—8 to 10 seconds.
Continue to work on overcoming blocks. Note also Exercise No. 17 for those who tend to waste time doing projects, watching TV or just never seeming to finish projects.

7. Complete journal entries.

WEEK SEVEN

It is now time in your imagery program to add exercises to **foster your special interests.** Rather than pick them out arbitrarily you can evaluate the kinds of imagery in the book that pertain to art, writing and drama and pick those that appeal to you.

You have tried 23 exercises in all, many of which have become part of your daily Exercise program. Certain ones like Meditation or the Inner Sanctuary serve special purposes to be used as desired. In the following weeks you will focus on areas of personal interest and become masters of creating your own imagery. Although I'll point out exercises that you should evaluate it is far more important to "get to know yourself" and focus on your dreams and aspirations that you want to realize. Your future is up for grabs. Grab it.

There are two final exercises that I believe everyone should try and consider using daily. Thereafter your selections will be personal.

1. **Exercise No. 30. Overcoming Creative Blocks by Role-playing**.

2. **Exercise No. 31. Assuming the Identity of a Master Artist**.

   This is for people interested in developing their artistic skills. The exercise works with painting, sculpture, pottery, woodwork and other artistic pursuits where a definable artist is recognized.

3. We now begin individual selectivity. Check out **Exercise No. 27. Write a Story**, **Exercise No. 28. Draw a Picture** and **Exercise No. 29. Creating a Drama**. All these exercises are written for group interactions, which you can try with your spouse, friends or other creative people.

   However, you can use those exercises strictly alone. Instead of depending on others to provide the stimulus, imagine that you are several people and write all the parts, or draw the entire picture or even play-act the roles in a drama. It's fun to try and by now you have become pretty knowledgeable about imagery and can easily maneuver into this creative area. Try it.

4. This week we're continuing the previous imagery only by now I imagine that most of you have made changes and have either added, modified or deleted some of your exercises.

6. Complete journal entries.

WEEK EIGHT

1. Continue your imagery exercises that are now strictly what currently work for you.
2. Today we'll tackle chronic or addictive behavior that affects many of us. One is overeating; another could be gambling or excessive drinking. Whatever problems you are struggling with try imagery to help you overcome them. In these cases you must absolutely believe in your desire

to get well. These types of compulsions are not easy to overcome but with a strong belief and will-power you can do it.

3. Evaluate **Exercise No. 39, 40 and 41. Controlling Compulsive Eating: The refrigerator, the cupboard and the dining table**.

> These three exercises for weight control are simple but very effective, when added to a diet program. Diet imagery is fun to construct since there are many possibilities based on what drives you to overeat.

4. **Exercise No. 36. Overcoming a Gambling Obsession.**

5. **Exercise No. 37. Inferiority and Gambling.**

6. **Exercise No. 38. Resolution of Gambling Compulsion**.

7. Complete journal entries.

WEEK NINE

1. Continue your imagery exercises.

2. This week you will create your own imagery. This will definitely be fun and will stimulate your **creative imagination**. Pick out three subjects that you want to focus on. They can be old or completely new areas. They can be directed to overcoming some problem or removing barriers. Don't hesitate to work over specific imagery exercises you already do that need improving.

   In the artistic world alone there are so many kinds of imagery that you can have a field day. Create imagery as preparation to try a new artistic pursuit. If you want to sing alone or join a choir but feel you sound hoarse or off-key practice singing and simultaneously create end-state imagery seeing yourself singing with a group or on stage.

People attempting to diet can really let loose with imagery that tackles every phase of their eating problem. Then there's imagery strictly for fun, such as creating stories in the mind or walking into imagery pictures and seeing where you go. Improve your golf swing or overhead tennis smash. There is absolutely no limit to your imagination. Be daring.

By now you should be gaining the benefits of imagery and have certainly opened up veins of fantasy and imagination.

3.   Complete your journal entries.

WEEK TEN

1. Continue your imagery.

2. Read over your journal and see the changes that you have noted as you progressed during the past ten weeks. See how you have overcome resistance and motivational problems. Note how you have changed and how you have used the journal. Evaluate how you can better use the journal. Some people make it more introspective, like an in-depth diary. Some use it to summarize their week's activities.

3. Go back into the cave or into a forest to again meet the wise person that you met in your first imagery exercise. Create another way to move into your inner world, such as flying to another planet or galaxy. Imagine different ways to know yourself. Create another you. Talk to animals. Visualize walking along a road and you meet someone as you round a bend in the road.

4. Complete your journal entries.

WEEK ELEVEN

1. Continue your imagery.

2. Imagine how you will enhance your romantic and sexual life. Reread chapters four, *Finding Romance* and five, *Igniting your Sex Life*, if needed.

3. As it is said. "You are what you believe." Believe in your ability to rise to previously unknown heights. See yourself as a giant in whatever areas you crave to excel. You are a giant. By now you can believe in your ability to focus on change and maintain the motivation and persistence to initiate those changes.

4. Complete your journal entries.

WEEK TWELVE

1. Continue your imagery.

2. This is your final week of growing younger and changing your life into a new and vital one. Think of what you have accomplished during these past three months. You have achieved a new way of thinking and living. There can be no doubt that you have gained much for your future based strictly upon your own mental power and belief in yourself. You followed a path not knowing initially where it would go.

3. I imagine that by now you're quite expert in developing imagery, new paths, finding new avenues of growth and discovering all sorts of exciting and fun activities, many of which you created in your mind. You have gone far beyond the simple exercises that you learned. Imagery is

only a beginning, a stimulus for change, a vehicle to provide the impetus for growth. You are a creative and vital person who wants to make this later time in your life as good as it gets. And you will, as the light of an exciting and new world shines on you.

Addendum No. 2

GUIDED IMAGERY

As a final exercise I have written a **guided imagery** exercise for all the young at heart. The best way to use this imagery is to record the entire exercise on an audio tape or CD or have someone read it to you. Then close your eyes and relax as you listen to it. Follow the words in your mind. Create the visual pictures. Hear the sounds. Immerse yourself in the fantasy. You can use this guided imagery whenever you want.

GUIDED IMAGERY EXERCISE

Sit in a comfortable chair. Close your eyes. Take several deep breaths and relax. Feel the tension leaving your body. You feel peaceful and know that you are about to go on a wonderful journey. Your mind opens to welcome whatever transpires. Visualize, hear and reflect on what is now to happen. Immerse yourself in the experience.

You're alone on a beach surrounded by cliffs. Soft clouds spread across the sky. Birds fly overhead. A tiny spotted sandpiper comes to land on your outstretched arm. You marvel at its trust. It looks directly into your eyes. So delicate and so beautiful. You gaze at it with wonderment. It slowly walks to your hand and gently picks at your fingers. After a final glance into your eyes the tiny bird flies off. You smile as you think how connected you felt to a creature of the wild for those few moments of time.

You walk on and reflect on how easily the tiny bird flew into the air. "I also can fly," you think. "I've been preparing for this special day. I want to fly. Fly into the sky. Fly to places of beauty. Fly into the unknown." With a sudden rush of excitement you know that today you can fly. And with no effort you soar into the sky. You are flying. You exult in the rush of air that caresses your body. Birds fly around you welcoming you into their midst. You marvel at your ability to do this and then realize that this is your time in life to fly to places never seen. This is your time to fly into a new world.

Ahead you see a luxuriant meadow filled with multi-colored wild flowers and surrounded by a forest of tall evergreen trees. You descend and walk among the flowers toward the forest. You bend down to smell a wild rose and gently reach out to entice a butterfly toward your hand. Again you smile and hug yourself for the welling up of a feeling of love for who you are and who you have become.

As you continue walking you feel something touch your leg and look down at the most beautiful white rabbit you have ever seen. His ears stand straight up and seem to tilt toward you. You stop and gaze into its soft brown eyes. Yes, there can be no mistake. The rabbit did smile at you even as it hopped into your arms to be held. You hold it tightly and watch in amazement as it falls asleep like a small child resting in its parent's arms. You walk on and suddenly hear the rustling of leaves and there in front of you is another rabbit and four baby rabbits. The rabbit in your arms awakens and reaches up to kiss you on your nose and then hops down and joins its family. The baby rabbits scamper around you wanting to be picked up and wanting to be caressed, which you do one at a time. After awhile they scamper away looking for seeds and nuts. You wave goodbye as you take leave of this loving family of rabbits.

You walk toward the forest noticing the flowers growing everywhere, butterflies flitting by, birds chattering away while sitting on the branches of trees. Two squirrels play tag and scurry by almost touching you. Inside the forest you are surrounded by the magnificent evergreen trees. You feel protected and reach out to touch a tree and feel its vibrations as it reacts to your touch. Deeply moved you hug it whispering of your love.

Again you take to the air and wonder if this is all a dream. Are you really flying? Did a tiny bird alight on your arm? Did you hold a beautiful rabbit in your arms? Even as you ponder the questions you are soaring through space and know that this is no dream. In wonderment you say convincingly, "I have changed into a person who can fly. The flying is in my mind. I can go anywhere and do anything. There are no limits. Limits don't exist for me."

With those thoughts you rise higher and higher into the sky. The earth recedes. You see clearly how truly beautiful the world is. As you look outward toward other planets and suns you know that the entire galaxy is within your reach. You are truly a part of this extraordinary universe.

Suddenly and impulsively, as part of your new freedom, you stop your ascent and dive toward the ocean far below. Within seconds you reach it and dive into its depths. You are not surprised that you can breathe underwater. As you descend to the ocean floor you are completely surrounded by colorful fish of all types and sizes.

Nearby is the opening of a great cave that you enter. The current pulls you along into the tunnels of the cave. On the walls you see pictures of astonishingly exquisite fish. Strange, exotic frogs hop by. Eels stretch out their long necks and gaze at you. Yellow and purple fish glide by and nibble at your ears. As you approach the center of the cave a large, magnificent dolphin swims toward you. A strangely, beautiful melody issues from its mouth and you gasp in astonishment realizing that you can understand its language.

The dolphin with a knowing look tells you that you have entered a magical world that will be forever open to you. The most exciting experiences await you as you reach further into your new world. The exploration of your new world is endless. You have truly become part of the living world even as you have become free within yourself.

As you ready to leave the cave the dolphin sings another song. It is a song of love, adventure, freedom and the connection to the world. The dolphin tells you to again fly high into the sky where you will experience the fullness of your new freedom. Now is the time to open your mind wider and wider. See your mind opening even now. Your mind will become as vast as the universe. "No limits. No limits," it chants.

Outside, you again take to the air. The planet below becomes smaller and smaller as you ascend. Ahead you see a shimmering halo that appears to be made of diffuse vapors. You feel excited as you approach and begin to enter the halo. And for a moment in time you are uplifted beyond words and feel a oneness with the spirit and the unity of the universe.

Once more you descend and enter a forest filled with ancient trees. Firs, spruces, poplars, cedars and sequoias surround you. You see tigers, elephants, squirrels, snakes, penguins, flamingoes, small robins, tiny chipmunks and countless other animals. All together. You marvel that so many different trees and animals are all in the same forest. You marvel as you realize that in this forest all trees and all creatures are equal and all are beautiful.

As you walk you ponder that being older is a blessing. You finally understand that you are a freer, more vital and happier person. And most of all you know that from your own mind has sprung all that you have experienced. You have become a creative, loving and bountiful person with love for all creatures and special love for yourself. It is now time to leave the forest and once more you soar into the sky.

Again you look down at the beauty of the earth swimming in the cosmos, unique and forever. Your love for your planet grips you. You love the land and the blue oceans that surround the continents. In a glance the grandness of the planet is spread before you. You realize that everything has coalesced. The rivers, the mountains, the deserts and the manmade edifices are part of the total beauty of the planet. All the countries throughout the earth are seen as one. The earth is one. You know that is what must be. A coming together of what nature and man has wrought. You are deeply moved by what you see and understand.

You are at peace and at one with the universe. Slowly, you glide back to earth until you are again sitting quietly in a chair with your eyes closed, feeling a deep tranquility and inner peacefulness. You saw the new you, the you that you had sought and have now become. You know that anytime you wish you can return to this wondrous world and reconnect to your universe. Open your eyes, smile and know that all is well in your life.

Addendum No. 3

INTRODUCTION TO MENTAL IMAGERY

Many opportunities await retirees as they enter their new world. To give you a new tool that could propel you forward at a faster and more exciting pace I'd like to introduce to you the power of mental imagery. I have used these techniques for many years helping people overcome negative beliefs, change unacceptable behavior, enhance creativity, maximize athletic skills, and develop healthy and joyful lifestyles.

The technique of mental imagery to change thinking and behavior has been around for hundreds of years. Sometimes called visualization or waking dreams, mental imagery is used in hypnosis, behavioral therapy, meditation, yoga and plain ordinary daydreaming.

Two famous musicians, Artur Rubinstein and Vladimir Horowitz resisted practicing the piano. Instead they would visualize playing entire concertos without physically moving a finger. The power of mental imagery was illustrated in the September 25, 2000 issue of Newsweek in the article "Olympic Mind Games." It reported how professional athletes, including Tiger Woods, Jack Nicklaus and Michael Jordan, utilize a strong mental imagery program to help develop prowess in their respective sports.

To better understand how imagery influences behavior and mental attitudes, let's enter the mind of a basketball player. To improve his shooting skills, a basketball player sits quietly with his eyes closed and imagines standing some predetermined distance from a basket. In minute detail, he visualizes his body posture, his arm movements, and the ball arching through the air on its way to the hoop. He visualizes making his movements as perfect as possible. The player practices mentally as part of his overall plan to maximize his skills.

Athletes can develop and improve their skills almost as effectively with imagery as with actual practice. However, to utilize the mental improvement of their skills, the athlete must go out on a court or field and practice in real time and in real action what he developed through imagery. In addition, he must do daily exercises, practice team coordination skills, and maintain a healthy body to compete. No athlete would become great only using imagery.

The same is true in most uses of imagery. The benefits accrue as the mental changes or new mindsets are used in actual activities to produce behavioral changes. By learning mental imagery techniques you will be able to develop a new set of beliefs and change your behavior in many areas of your life. In almost all endeavors you may undertake, mental imagery could be used as a facilitator. You can eradicate negative beliefs and modify misperceptions. People entering their senior years are especially eager to make changes in their lives in order to make this period fruitful and happy. And they have time to put to use whatever they learn.

For example, if you have decided that now is the time to attempt to reach your desired weight then mental imagery can help as a part of a diet. Overweight people, who practice imagery exercises, can change how they eat, when they eat and their feelings about their body. You can overcome compulsive eating.

You can foster many other changes to enhance your life. You can visualize becoming an artist or a writer or a better golfer. You can improve your sex life. Your imagination will help determine what kinds of imagery will best suit your wishes and endeavors.

Belief Systems or Mindsets:

Belief systems or mindsets involve mental attitudes that determine who we are, how we function as human beings, what we do, how we treat ourselves, how we treat others, and even how we treat the world we live in. Belief systems are positive, negative, or neutral.

Positive beliefs include high self-esteem, loving yourself and others, feeling that you are loved and admired, trusting yourself, knowing that you are creative and productive, and that you enjoy sharing your knowledge. Having the belief in your own integrity and ability to control your life is one that governs most other beliefs. If you believe you can achieve your goals, that positive belief will guide you toward them.

Negative beliefs include low self-esteem, excessive guilt over anger, shame about your body, doubt regarding your intelligence, diminished capacity to work efficiently and accepting any negative attitude about yourself. If you believe you are incapable of attaining your goals, that negative belief will thwart you. Other powerful negative beliefs include believing that you cannot consciously control your behavior and that an inner force or compulsion makes you act as you do. These negative beliefs often give rise to self-condemnation, guilt over unacceptable behavior, depression, feelings of inferiority, and self-hate.

Neutral beliefs have little to do with conscious actions, but rather deal with unconscious or autonomous behavior. An example would be walking. We take for granted that we can walk without exerting conscious control over our movements. But even the ability to walk can be changed. Under hypnosis a person can be made to believe that he can no longer move his legs and he can't walk. His inner belief has changed. Such behavioral change can also occur from fear. Being "rooted to the spot" or "paralyzed with fear" are common sayings that reveal our belief that our ability to walk can be changed.

The Power of Beliefs

We all take for granted that we can't fly. But in dreams we become believers and easily fly. Sometimes in the awake state a delusion overcomes reality, and a person believing he can fly may fling himself from a rooftop. Beliefs are powerful tools of the mind. They can operate for good or for bad. You are going to learn constructive beliefs.

Types of Imagery

We think of imagery as primarily visual. However, other sensory elements, such as smell, taste, body movements, and sound are frequently present in the imagery. Through one's imagination a picture is projected onto a visual screen. Such images can then be utilized for various purposes to change mindsets and behavior.

IMAGERY CAN BE DIVIDED INTO FOUR TYPES:

Literal Imagery

Images that realistically represent the object used in the visualization. For example, a realistic looking heart.

Symbolic Imagery

Images that are suggestive in appearance or action of the object considered for visualization. For example, a large metal mechanical pump that represents a heart.

Process Imagery

A series of literal or symbolic images that represent an activity, a changing procedure, or a continuous process. For example, visualizing the movement of food through the body starting with the mouth and ending in the colon. This would comprise a series of distinct, though connected, images.

End State Imagery

Images that represent the final state of a desired process. For example, seeing yourself being able to paint beautiful pictures or be in excellent physical condition or, if on a diet, seeing yourself at your ideal weight.

THE PLAN FOR CREATING YOUR IMAGERY PROGRAM:

1. Decide what mindset and/or behavior pattern you want to change.
2. Choose the imagery setting that represents where your specific problem takes place. Imagery settings are simply the visual descriptions of the place, venue, emotional state, or situation that describes what you want to change.
3. Decide on the imagery that will help you combat the specific problem presented in that setting.
4. Determine an affirmation that will emphasize and strengthen your resolve to change.

THREE EXAMPLES TO ILLUSTRATE HOW AN IMAGERY EXERCISE IS DEVELOPED:

1. **Mindset**: Belief that you are a writer with writer's block. The imagery setting can be one of many. The block may occur when you sit down at your typewriter or computer or when you are trying to create or imagine a topic to write about. Or each time you start to write you are overwhelmed with a need to sleep. You would then create the imagery to combat these various behaviors.

The imagery setting: You are sitting at the typewriter seeing your hands frozen in place (a symbolic version of writer's block).

Imagery to change behavior: Look at your frozen hands and say to yourself that frozen hands will no longer be part of your body. With those words a piercing beam of light comes out of your mind and instantly thaws your hands. Your fingers immediately start to rapidly type. Your fertile mind accompanies the movement of your fingers, as idea after idea pours forth, resulting in continuous typing.

A simple affirmation might be: I have the mental power to overcome my writer's block or I will never suffer from writer's block again. You say this to yourself at the end of the imagery. See below.

There are many settings and exercises to fight writer's block dependent only on your imagination.

To be effective, imagery is exaggerated and an intense emotion governs the exercise. You also believe in what you are imagining and in your mental power to change your behavior. The imagery helps create a new belief system to diminish or even eradicate the unacceptable thoughts and behavior.

2. **Mindset:** Believing you are overweight and thus unattractive (see below for additional diet imagery).

The imagery setting: Seeing yourself as excessively heavy and starting a diet. You could visualize a dining room table filled with your favorite foods and feeling overwhelmed by a powerful wish to binge. You visualize yourself reaching for the food.

Imagery to change behavior: Overcoming the tendency to binge on food on a dining table can be as simple as waving your hand in a magical gesture and making the food disappear in a cloud of smoke or turning the food into something obnoxious and thus inedible. If you want to be even more daring and are not offended by highly unpleasant images, which can be very powerful, you can imagine a large ax descending from above, as you reach for food that cuts off your hands. Any of these images would complete the imagery exercise.

Affirmation: I will never binge on food from a dining table again.

3. **Mindset**: Feeling painful inferiority or suffering from strong self-doubt and self-criticism or undue passivity that stymies your efforts to change your behavior.

The imagery setting: If you were filled with self-doubt or inferiority, you could visualize yourself torn with conflict, perhaps shrunken in size or your head could be bursting with pain or you are shaking with anguish until your body feels like it's flying apart. That would constitute the imagery setting.

Imagery to change the emotional state: You could combat this belief by suddenly seeing yourself expand and become a giant and feel great power and belief in yourself. Or a brilliant white light can enclose your body and immediately change your negative beliefs. You become whole and the master of your life and future. The white light disappears and a totally confident you remains.

Affirmation: I will never again feel self-doubt about myself or my abilities. The power of my mind will overcome any such doubts.

You select imagery that fits your symptoms. The mind always knows the intent of the procedure and the exact imagery is less important than your strong belief in what you are doing and its effectiveness. Your imagination is unlimited.

The imagery can be modified, changed, or combined. New ones can be added. Old ones can be eliminated. You may think of some others that will fit your needs. You will determine the continuing usefulness of whatever imagery you decide on.

Practice the imagery exercises daily for weeks or months, or until you have overcome the unacceptable behavior. Imbue the imagery with as much feeling as possible. The imagery works because you want to change your unacceptable behavior. You want the imagery to work. You are opening your mind to your own suggestions, because you want to write freely and creatively or change eating patterns. Imagery works because you have faith that your mind can control your behavior. Mental imagery is a creative and dynamic method that can effectively modify thinking and behavior patterns.

THE PRACTICE OF IMAGERY

Imagery is best practiced in a state of deep relaxation. You can use any relaxation technique you wish, such as meditation, progressive relaxation, or deep breathing. The technique that I have used for many years is quick and effective and can be accomplished in the space of two deep breaths. Do not practice this technique while in a car.

The Rag Doll Technique:

Sit in a comfortable chair. Relax your body. Close your eyes. Visualize yourself as a rag doll. To enhance this visual picture it may help to shake your arms and legs a few moments in a loose manner like a rag doll.

Take a slow, deep breath. As you slowly exhale, imagine pouring your mental self into your rag doll self. Take another slow, deep breath and again slowly exhale and once more pour your mental self into your rag doll self. You are now in a deep state of relaxation.

Practice the rag doll technique a few times until you are comfortable with it, and can truly feel the deep relaxation that is conducive to practicing the imagery exercises.

For those who desire to gauge the timing of your breathing, count to four on inhaling, hold your breath to the count of two and then exhale to the count of four. As soon as you feel comfortable with the rate of your breathing, there is no need to count.

Starting your Imagery Program:

To start your program, determine what thoughts and behavior you wish to modify or eliminate and create your imagery, as described above. Most conditions can generally benefit from multiple imagery exercises and I suggest you start with three or four. In general, all imagery programs should include one end-state exercise that shows you as you want to be when you have overcome the unwanted behavior.

Example: Many older people suffer from anxiety when they meet strangers or face groups. There are many possible imagery exercises to combat this condition. The following four imagery exercises are typical examples.

1. **Visualize walking into a room of strangers** who appear very angry, distant, and unfriendly. You are extremely

anxious.   To overcome the resultant stress you imagine yourself warm and open, and totally at ease. You go over to each person, no matter how unfriendly they appear and introduce yourself. Each person quickly warms up to you and is obviously pleased to meet you. You see yourself speaking with confidence and ease. You say emphatically that you will never be afraid to reach out to strangers again.

2. **A variation of the previous exercise**. Imagine entering a room filled with strangers who are indifferent to you. You feel ignored and disliked. You immediately act very positive and outgoing and quietly exude confidence and warmth. People turn to you in a very friendly manner and make it clear they like you immensely. You say to yourself with great conviction that you are a loving and caring person, and people will always like you much as you like and love yourself.

3. **Here is an example of a somewhat different imagery exercise** where the anxiety is more akin to fear of being hurt or ridiculed. You are walking on a street feeling very small and fearful. People stare at you and call you names and spit on you. You decide that you are no longer going to tolerate being abused, ridiculed, or intimidated by anyone. You watch yourself grow taller and become a giant, either physically, mentally, or both. With great vigor and power you tell all those who were abusing you that you will no longer tolerate their abuse. They will stop or you will destroy them. You say to yourself that you have now become a powerful person and nothing or no one will ever frighten or abuse you again.

4. **Create one of your exercises as end-state imagery**. Visualize walking into a room crowded with strangers. You are totally at ease, smiling, reaching out, and introducing yourself to person after person. Everyone obviously enjoys your friendly and warm manner and responds with similar feelings. You walk into other places where you are totally confident.   Everyone   greets   you.   You   make   easy conversation and people want to be around you. You feel

good, knowing you can now reach out to care for anyone you desire. Nothing will ever thwart you again.

Other Ways to Develop and Use Imagery:

Example: Since dieting is frequently on the minds of overweight seniors, it's frequently valuable to incorporate mental imagery into your diet program.

An overweight person seeks to gain permanent weight control. Dependent on what kinds of situations stimulate the overeating, this person could develop the following imagery exercises.

1. Open the refrigerator door to get food for binging. Out jumps an enormous rat (or other animal or insect) attempting to bite you (negative imagery). You back away and say loudly and convincingly that you will never again use the refrigerator for binging.

2. See a dining table filled with your favorite foods that you reach for. All the food immediately turns inedible or into ferocious animals that bite your hand, which immediately makes you back away again saying that you will never reach for food for binging from a table. Or as soon as you see the tempting food, you sweep it to the floor in one swift movement saying you will never let food tempt you again.

3. See yourself at your ideal weight, walking down the street being admired by people, and/or seeing yourself in a bathing suit at the beach in your desired body size, in excellent physical shape, seeing yourself run along the beach without difficulty, feeling good about your new body and knowing others are admiring you (end-state imagery).

Most imagery is very simple and thus may seem ineffective. Nothing could be further from the truth. Your mind knows your intent and believing in what you do is sufficient to make the changes. It makes no difference how you construct your imagery as long as you believe it fits your specific problem. You are trying to overcome a deficiency with mental power and your mind listens.

Most people experiment extensively during the first few weeks. Rarely do the first imagery exercises remain constant throughout their program. Even when the initial imagery fits the problem, it's apt to be modified as experience with imagery grows. Above all, try to be as creative as possible and enjoy developing it. And always exaggerate the imagery. The greater the emotional reaction the better. Within a week or two you will have created a useful program that fits your particular needs. These exercises will become an important part of your continuing desire for increased well-being and self-control.

Your emotional state, while engaged in your imagery program, should include high self-esteem, exuberance, and joy in your new sense of well-being. Even if you are in a state of depression or self-doubt, visualize rising above those feelings when you do the imagery.

When creating the end-state imagery you must believe that you will reach your goal. The belief is what feeds your auto-suggestibility and creates the matrix for changes in your thinking and behavior. Even if you have trouble fully believing in the power of imagery at first, make believe that you do.

Timing and Frequency

Try to do the full program, i.e. all your imagery exercises, at least three times a day and, if possible, as much as 20 times a day. With imagery, more is better. Frequently, ten to twenty seconds per exercise is sufficient. Thus, a program with five or six different exercises may only take a few minutes. Experiment with doing the full program of exercises more frequently, alternating with shorter periods, until you determine what feels best. Some people prefer to repeat certain exercises for several minutes rather than go over a number of exercises. Trust your judgment. Practice and experiment until you find that combination of exercises and time that works for you. The benefits of these exercises will become evident.

HOW DOES MENTAL IMAGERY WORK?

Although the exact way mental imagery works is not known, there are a number of things about it that we do understand. It is primarily a visualization technique using the power of autosuggestion. The fact that it influences us is no longer questioned. Self-induced mental imagery works through repetition and by directing its effect upon existing beliefs or mindsets. These beliefs can be changed.

Recent studies show the physiological effect of imagery on brain functions. Visualization studies of Ian Robertson of Trinity College, Dublin, and Stephen Kosslyn of Harvard University show that visualization activates many of the same areas of the brain that actual physical activity does. When you imagine throwing a basketball into a hoop with deep concentration while sitting quietly in a chair, as in our previous illustration, the same neuronal circuits and brain areas are affected as though you were engaged in the activity on a real basketball court.

PET (Positron Emission Topography) scans and functional MRI studies show that mental imagery produces similar physical changes in the brain whether the activity is real or imagined. The effect is just as permanent with the imagery as with the actual activity.

Imagery is related to night dreams. Apparently, images in the mind, especially symbolic ones, tap into the unconscious and thus become linked to deep internal elements in our inner self. Thus, imagery taps the power of the unconscious, as well as the conscious mind.

In a state of relaxation, sometimes understood as an alpha state, the mind is very open and susceptible to autosuggestion. By using mental imagery, you are directly influencing yourself. You become your own teacher. You gradually give up any influences from the outside world and from your own negative belief systems. The stronger you desire to change and the more firmly you believe in the imagery technique the more likely you will be influenced by what you think. When you couple a strong desire and belief to an effective technique, you will have achieved a way of processing imagery to change your mindsets and behavior.

The most Important Elements in the use of Mental Imagery:

- Believe in the power of your mind to change your behavior.

- Believe in the technique of mental imagery to induce these changes.

- Maintain a strong and unwavering desire to overcome your negative mindsets and unacceptable behavior.

- Never falter in the repetition of the imagery. Changes do not occur with a few brief imagery exercises. Ask the athletes who use it with great devotion. They will practice for hours each day for many weeks or months to accomplish what they desire. The technique of using mental power to change oneself has been used for centuries. There's no magic. It's strictly understanding and using the techniques until you have gained your desired goals.

Most thought patterns can be changed. The belief in your ability to use your mind to make these changes by using a proven technique, such as mental imagery, makes it possible. By practicing these techniques you can eradicate negative mindsets and allow new ones to take their place.

To be successful the cardinal rule of any self-help program must be followed. **That rule is—maintain motivation**. The process helps you change the way you think, the way you act and react, and the way you live. Motivation is easier to maintain at the outset, since you have high hopes and a strong desire to change. The challenge is to maintain that motivation, start to finish.

But, if you begin to sense that motivation is slipping, examine your resistances and especially evaluate any negative feelings about what you are doing. Not believing fully in the power of mental imagery can diminish, if not eliminate, its effectiveness.

Intensify your Motivation with the Following Ideas:

1.   Believe in the value of mental imagery even if you have had no prior experience with it. It has been repeatedly demonstrated that each of us has an enormous, yet virtually untapped, capacity for taking control of our minds. Mental imagery is one of the most frequently used tools for facilitating this process.

2.   Stir up a powerful feeling of desire to change your behavior. Make a list of the things you dislike most about your life and another list of ways in which change will enhance your life. Keep adding to the lists. Keep reading and rereading them. Our minds tend to forget things that are inconvenient or painful to remember.

3.   Share your desire to change with those closest to you. Once you go public with your commitment, your friends, family and associates will become your strongest support team. Avoid any naysayer. Many people prefer to exercise their new mental control in private and feel that sharing is of little value. Evaluate and go with your feelings.

4. Exercise patience. Do not stop until you have changed your mindset about the behavior you desire to modify. Practice the mental imagery exercises as long as necessary in order to reach the desired goal. Your ability to succeed starts and ends with motivation.

5. Creating imagery offers many people an exciting method for self-exploration, developing insight, and expanding self-esteem. You have hidden resources that can be tapped by stimulating your creative imagination. You can attain a level of vitality and well-being that may once have seemed out of reach. Most importantly, you have a new tool to help

you realize your dreams and discover the path to a happier and more fulfilling life.

ABOUT THE AUTHOR

As a retiree himself, Marvin H. Berenson, M.D. has retained a perpetual sense of youthfulness and aliveness. He has lived an exciting life and an even more exciting retirement.

During many years of clinical practice and teaching, Dr. Berenson gained an enormous understanding of the human condition. For the last twenty years of his practice he specifically focused on mature adults acquiring much additional knowledge and insight about this rich and varied time period. Opening a new world to retirees became his passion.

Dr. Berenson saw the need for a book for older people that would encompass the ideas, mental imagery techniques and exercises that he has successfully used to enhance creativity, improve artistic and literary skills, help athletes maximize their performances and treat various physical and emotional problems. And so *Loving Life in Retirement* came into being. It fits precisely into his belief that people can change their thinking and behavior by following certain guidelines.

Dr. Berenson has a lifelong interest in creativity, mental imagery, sexual behavior, spirituality and holds a firm belief that no one should live life unfulfilled or stymied by inner or outer obstacles. He has devoted his life to helping many people overcome barriers freeing them to lead happy and meaningful lives.

He watched as people grew and flourished. He is convinced that by knowing how to overcome negative mindsets people are capable of changing how they think and how they live. If they want to change, change is ahead. They only need to know the techniques and methods to pursue a new path.

Dr. Berenson is Clinical Professor Emeritus of Psychiatry at the USC Keck School of Medicine and has been a Training and Supervising Analyst with the Los Angeles Society and Institute of Psychoanalysis. He is a member of the American Psychiatric Association, the American Psychoanalytic Association, the International Psychoanalytic Association, and the Alpha Omega Alpha Honorary Medical Society.

He lives with his wife, Irene, in Palos Verdes Estates, California. Together they share the love and friendship of six children and ten grandchildren. Among his many interests are writing, painting, sculpting, composing, gardening, hiking, reading, movies, playing the synthesizer and drums, play-acting and surfing the Internet.

www.ingramcontent.com/pod-product-compliance
Lightning Source LLC
Chambersburg PA
CBHW072111270326
41931CB00010B/1527